All Clear

All Clear

❧ An Everyday Guide to Total Skin Care

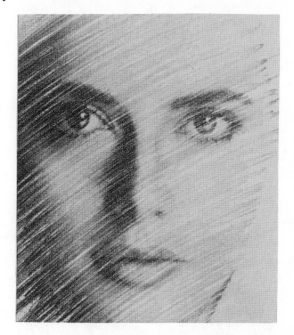

Treila Krueger

Betterway Publications, Inc.

First Printing: September, 1984

Published by Betterway Publications, Inc.
White Hall, VA 22987

Book design by Diane Nelson
Illustrations by Cynthia Burke
Typography by East Coast Typography, Inc.

Library of Congress Cataloging in Publication Data

Krueger, Treila
  All clear.

  Includes index.
  1. Skin—Care and hygiene.   I. Title.
RL87.K78   1984   616.5'05   84-12502
ISBN 0-932620-39-6 (pbk.)

Printed in the United States of America.

Dedicated to my lovely grandmother,
Ethel Adamson Tidwell

ABOUT THE AUTHOR

Treila Krueger lives in Northern California, holds a Master's Degree from the University of Texas and has done post graduate work at the University of California. As a nutritionist and preventive health care consultant, she is involved with the development of individual and institutional health care programs.

During her affiliation with the Children's Hospital in Bogota, Colombia, she developed preventive health care strategies for university-level hospitals. This research was published by Academic Press/Society of Community Medicine, London, England. Her extensive travels throughout this country and abroad have enabled her to study the health, nutrition, and skin care practices of women from varying cultural backgrounds and age groups.

In addition to her work as a nutritionist and preventive health care consultant, Treila teaches classes in nutrition, skin care, and make-up application. She also conducts group and individual sessions on these subjects for a cosmetic company.

Contents

Author's Note

This book is not meant to be a treatise on skin care, but was conceived primarily as a preventive skin care guide for all women. An attempt has been made to avoid highly technical terminology so that the reader may follow and understand the subject.

No specific time formula for a skin care regimen has been presented as individual needs vary and since the skin care process itself is an ever-changing, lifelong concern. The basic principles and techniques underlying effective skin care, however, are applicable to women of all ages, and must be practiced regularly for long-lasting results.

To help the reader distinguish between different types of cosmetic products, various brand names have been mentioned throughout the book. Such brands have been chosen on the basis of quality, price, and availability; and there are several other effective brands as well. Since individuals respond differently to various products, it is very difficult to recommend a particular name brand for everyone. Read the labels carefully before purchasing and always perform a patch test as suggested by the manufacturer.

For those who are affected by a particular skin problem such as acne or skin allergies, it is advisable to work in consultation with a dermatologist.

❧ ACKNOWLEDGMENTS

I wish to express my deep appreciation to all of those who contributed to the development of this book. I would especially like to convey my gratitude to:

Jacqueline and Robert Hostage, my publishers, for their excellent help, advice, and enthusiasm from day one;

Suresh K. Aery for his thoughtful editorial guidance;

Nancy Page, M.D. for her review of the manuscript;

Ramah Wokoun for sharing her knowledge and experience in the field of skin care;

My mother for her encouragement and interest in this project;

Cathy Wood for her patience and devotion to the project;

Patty O'Connor for her excellent secretarial assistance;

Suzan Browning for preparing the original cover design.

Grateful acknowledgment is made for permission to reprint the following:

Formula F Plus, page 129.
From *Swedish Beauty Secrets*
By Paavo O. Airola
(Phoenix, AZ: Health Plus Publishers, 1982)

Introduction

I have observed women of all ages and classes seeking more information in the area of skin care. "Which products are the *best* ones? How can I improve the appearance of my face?" or "I take good care of my skin but my problems won't go." After searching bookstores for comprehensive information on skin care, I found a number of books written by actresses or models, a few by salon specialists, and even fewer by dermatologists. However, almost all of these books advocate a particular solution: Dietary changes *will* improve your skin, facial exercise will bring about a more youthful appearance, the "right" cosmetics and dermatological treatments will remove years from your face. Nowhere did I locate a book that treated the subject of skin health in an integrated manner, focusing on the many personal, environmental, and commercial elements affecting the health and beauty of one's skin.

From personal experience I know that women want straightforward information on skin care practices and preservation. Many highly technical books are available which provide only the theory of skin care, but what women really want to know is how to acquire and maintain healthy, attractive skin without investing in ineffective or time-consuming techniques. They want to side-step rip-offs and learn how to develop integrated approaches to skin care. This book is offered not to promote any particular techniques, products, or procedures, but to bring together in simple, everyday language the most important elements of skin care practice and preservation.

The vast cache of knowledge in chemistry, biology, and other medical sciences is yet to be fully utilized in the field of skin and beauty care products. However, manufacturers in this field, as in other industries, are heavily oriented toward maximizing profits, consequently, many "new" products continue to appear that are often almost identical to those produced years, if not decades earlier. For example, the standard cold cream formula was discovered centuries ago by a Greek physician named Galen. The original formula consisted of a mixture of beeswax, olive oil, water and rose petals. Today "cold cream" is marked under a great number of names at a large price range. The basic formula is still being used, but olive oil has been replaced by other oils which do not become rancid as easily.

Women invest a great deal of money on widely advertised skin care products and techniques, many of which are extremely overpriced, time-consuming, and misleading in the claims they make. In this on-going pursuit of beauty, women continue to search for new products that might be more effective than older ones. The result is attractive packaging, advertising, and marketing of many old products with new names.

Cosmetic manufacturers must deal with complex problems such as product preparation, preservation, and transportation, and most money is spent on improvements in these areas, rather than in research that could possibly result in truly improved beauty solutions. Of course, not all existing products are near replicas of those used in earlier times. There have been some significant improvements in the quality and usefulness of many beauty care products. But even with such advances, it is often difficult to choose from the vast selection of existing products.

To challenge any practice or segment of the health or beauty industries is not the purpose of this book. Rather, one important aim is to direct the reader through the multitude of skin care products and techniques so that she might select the ones most beneficial to her own skin and avoid those products that are inappropriate. It will introduce her to the basic cosmetic ingredients and techniques and aid her in assessing their effectiveness and impact on her skin.

Knowing how to achieve and maintain radiant, healthy skin is an acquired skill that calls for practice and specialized knowledge. No one product, method, or technique can be right for every face. But the underlying factors that can make or break a healthy face are universal. Such factors include the basic facial regimen, practice of good nutrition and healthy lifestyle habits, control over personal, environmental, and seasonal elements affecting the skin's condition, selection and application of suitable skin care products, proper make-up selection and removal, utilization of special maintenance techniques, and sufficient rest and relaxation. The skin care process need not be a complicated, expensive, or time-consuming task. At the same time, there is not a single miracle product or technique available. In fact, the key to making the most of one's facial attributes lies not in wasting time chasing widely advertised products, techniques, or single-approach beauty plans, but in practicing consistently an appropriate and integrated skin care regimen. With the practical information provided in this book, the skin-conscious woman will be able to design her own skin care programs without getting lost in the ever-expanding jungle of health and beauty products and techniques.

1. The Skin:
What it is and How it works

As the largest organ of the human body, skin is composed of billions of organic cells and carries out many vital functions. It protects the body as a whole from bacteria and infection and shields internal organs from the sun's ultraviolet rays and from invasion by other foreign matter. The skin also aids in the elimination of waste material through perspiration, and it is sensitive to pain and pleasure from the outside environment. Although the skin is a protective external organ, it is greatly affected by the functioning of other parts of the body. This means that in order for the skin to function well it must not be impaired by a lack of nutrients or oxygen, extensive stress, disease or any prolonged internal dysfunction.

Three layers make up the skin — the epidermis, dermis, and fatty layer. The epidermis is the top layer that is outwardly visible. It serves as a shield to the dermis and is composed of two parts: the inner part directly beneath the dermis called the stratum Malpighii and an outer section of horny cells called the stratum corneum. In the stratum Malpighii, there is a basal layer of cells that provides continuous cell reproduction for the entire epidermis. As new cells are formed, they work their way to the skin's surface and there is a marked increase in the amount of keratin (a cell-manufactured protein substance) within the cells. When they reach the outer layer of the epidermis, they are dead cells composed entirely of keratin. Cells continue to grow, develop, die, and dry out through a process called keratinization. If there is too little or even too much keratin

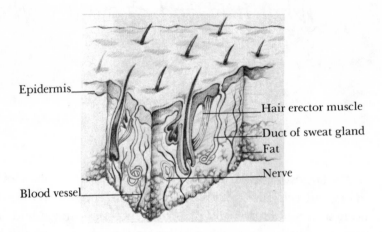

Epidermis

Hair erector muscle

Duct of sweat gland

Fat

Nerve

Blood vessel

formation, or if the keratinization occurs at a very abnormal speed, problems such as skin cracking, thickening, and flaking occur. For the keratin to remain healthy, the skin must contain an abundant supply of water. If there is a shortage of moisture in your skin, the keratin dries, and the cells break up. The result is dry skin.

As these dead cells accumulate on the outer layer of your skin, they should be removed. The process of removing dead cells is often referred to as sloughing or exfoliation and should be practiced daily to stimulate new cell growth in the underlying layers and to improve the appearance of your skin. If you've ever wondered why your complexion appears muddled and dull, it's probably because too many dead cells have built up on the outer surface of the epidermis. Such buildup of waste materials not only affects growth of future cells, it plugs up your pores and leads to the formation of blackheads and pimples.

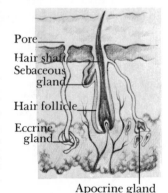

Pore

Hair shaft

Sebaceous gland

Hair follicle

Eccrine gland

Apocrine gland

On the skin's outer surface, there is an acid mantle made up primarily of water and oil from the sweat and sebaceous glands. This fluid coating the outside layer of skin serves as a natural moisturizer and protects the skin from any type of pollution or infection. The natural pH of human skin (measurement of skin acidity) is between 4.5 - 5.5. And although there are individual variations, 5.5 is generally considered the average. To maintain a healthy acid mantle, (the filmy fluid coating the top skin) it is necessary to choose products compatible with your skin's acidity. For most people, this means selecting a neutral or mildly acidic product and soaps that are not highly alkaline. The skin's texture can be further upset by harsh soap products or consistent use of cosmetic formulas which are highly acidic.

Although skin problems are often visible on the epidermis, many of them begin below the skin's surface in the dermal layer. The dermis supports the epidermis and contains nerve endings, oil and sweat glands, fat cells, blood and lymph vessels, and hair follicles. Within the dermis is also a network of fibers, known as connective tissues and composed primarily of a protein called collagen. This collection of fibers provides your skin with strength, form, and resilience. As long as the collagen network is strong, smooth, and pliable, your skin will appear youthful and firm. But when the fibers become inflexible and disorganized with age, the skin begins to sag and wrinkle.

Age alone, however, is not the only factor that promotes the break up of your collagen fibers. Often, too much sun, prolonged illness, nutritional deficiency and pollution, including cigarette smoke, can impair the condition of this collagen network. The genetic factor also impacts these connective tissues and their ability to withstand abuse and the test of time. Whatever the causes may be, the damage or loss of this important underlying structure will result in wrinkled and aged skin.

It is clear that what happens within the dermal layer directly affects the health and beauty of the epidermis. If the skin's outside layer is to stay healthy, the inside layers must be properly nourished. Even though an aging structure within the skin cannot be restored, there are preventive measures such as proper nutrition and regular exercise, avoidance of chemicals and pollution and overexposure to sun that can at least provide insurance against premature aging.

The third layer of skin below the dermis is the subskin. This section is made up of fatty and muscle tissue and serves to protect the top skin as well as the whole body from heat and cold, bacterial infection or internal damage. Again, the condition of this layer affects the outer skin's appearance. What you can do to keep this part healthy is maintain a balanced diet combined with a vigorous exercise program.

2. Assessing and Caring for your Skin

❧ SKIN ANALYSIS

Before applying cleansers, make-up, masques, moisturizers, or any type of cosmetic product, you must take stock of your present skin type. Since facial skin is constantly changing due to both environmental and biological factors, it's absolutely vital that you keep up-to-date on the state of your skin. At age thirty-five, for example, you wouldn't want to be using the same products you used at twenty-one. As the skin's texture and appearance gradually change, you should adapt your skin care practices accordingly.

In order to discover your true skin type or update your skin analysis, you'll need to think back a bit to study the history of your skin, your parents' skin type, the color of your hair and your complexion. Each of these factors influences your skin's conditions throughout all phases of life. To analyze your skin accurately, here are two simple tests that you can perform.

Test # 1

Clean your skin thoroughly. Take a large hand mirror and in direct morning sunlight, spot check each area of the face for oily or dry patches. Repeat the process twice.

Test # 2

About 15-45 minutes after rising in the morning, rub a piece of paper from a grocery bag across your forehead. (Before cleansing the skin). If your skin in that area is about normal, the paper will turn slightly darker. If the paper is translucent to the point where you can see through it more easily than before rubbing, your skin is oily. The more soaked the paper, the oilier your skin. If the paper retains its original color, your skin is probably a bit too dry. Check all other areas of your face via the same process. Remember that dry skin becomes more apparent in colder weather, while oily skin will show up more in warm and humid climates.

If you are still unsure as to what type skin you have, the following skin-type characteristics will help you decide.

Oily Skin Characteristics

1. Your face begins to "shine" a few hours or even sooner after make-up application.
2. Your hair is oily and must be washed almost every day to look healthy.
3. During adolescence you suffered from acne and following this period (after 21) your pimples continued, although the condition was less severe than before.
4. Your face tends to absorb make-up and/or there is uneven coverage. Your skin may be oily in some areas, normal or even dry in others, thereby creating problems with even make-up coverage.
5. Your skin tends to easily attract debris of all kinds and you find that it needs washing more frequently than twice a day.
6. The nose, chin, and forehead tend to remain somewhat oily in some women during the mid-twenties and beyond. If any or all of these areas appear greasy, then your skin is too oily.
7. In adults, dandruff and continued acne problems may also indicate an oily skin condition.

Dry Skin Characteristics

1. Lines and wrinkles become more visible in dry skin — especially across the forehead and under the eyes. Do you have signs of lines and wrinkles even though you are still in your twenties or thirties?

2. Does your skin tone appear dull, with fine pores?
3. Does your skin appear flaky, chapped or cracked?

Normal Skin Characteristics _____

1. If your skin is normal, you may expect that a make-up base will remain fairly attractive-looking even at the end of the day — without shininess, cracking, or uneven color showing through.
2. If you can go days without using creams and masques and your skin is still soft, smooth, and glowing, the skin is probably normal.
3. Do your parents have healthy skin — free of acne and excess oil? Do you have very few, if any enlarged pores? Does your hair remain reasonably attractive after two or three days without washing?
4. Does your skin respond well to creams and lotions after exposure to sun or cold weather, you have a fairly clear complexion now, and had very mild acne as an adolescent?

Once you have learned your basic skin type, you should follow the *five steps* listed below in order to develop and maintain a lovely facial skin and to reduce the negative effects of aging, environmental pollution and any other culprits that might negatively affect your skin. These five basic steps include:*

1. Make-up removal and cleansing
2. Granular scrubbing and exfoliation
3. Toning
4. Moisturizing/Nourishing
5. Stimulating

* Each step discussed in detail in this chapter and the following one.

♣ *HOW TO CARE FOR OILY SKIN*

An oily skin is very common among adolescents in the 14-21 year cycle and is much easier to control than dry skin. There's no need to apply cream and moisturizers to oily skin at this age as it produces plenty of its own oil naturally. Adding oily products to adolescent skin will cause more harm than good. Oily skin or patches of oiliness, also exist in adult women, although oily skin at this stage occurs as a result of varying influences. Factors affecting oily skin include environmental elements (intense humidity stimulates oil production and chemicals polluting the air may do the same) and hormonal imbalances. Overindulging in certain foods may also affect the condition of skin in some people. Although there is no real proof that food elements per se will induce oiliness, heavy reliance on certain food elements may aggravate oily skin. Finally, you may inherit a tendency toward oily skin.

Oily skin is usually accompanied by many enlarged pores that contain blackheads (A blackhead is a plug of oil which has reacted with oxygen on the surface and turned black). The skin, if very oily, will often have an unhealthy yellowish tint. In general, the oiliness is caused by an overproduction of sebum (oil) by the sebaceous glands. (oil glands); blackheads usually result when this excess production of oil occurs. The pore channels which are filled with oil combine with air and oxidize, turning brownish-black in appearance. The black represents oxidized oil, not dirt from the outside. Poor cleansing habits, pollution, dead cells, and make-up debris make the problem even worse.

Make-Up Removal and Cleansing

Ideally, you should clean your face with a soap or facial cleanser designed for oily skin. The best and worst of facial cleansers are much more expensive than a bar of soap but if your budget allows, a foam or liquid cleanser can be effective. Here again, it helps to know your skin well so that you can avoid buying a product that you are allergic to or that is otherwise unsuitable. If you choose soap as your method of cleansing, the soap should be a bit stronger than those designed for other skin types. Do not just buy any sweet-smelling detergent soap at your local market. Your best bet is to read the labels carefully and select a soap for oily skin that contains very little, if any, tar, sulphur, resorcinol, and salicylic acid. Choose a product that is low in alcohol as well. For oily skin combined with acne, your choice of soap should include one that is designed especially for acne. Cleansing grains developed for oily and acned skin include Brasivol and Pernox. Komex and Fostex are additional cleansing agents that you might consider. Buff Puff may also be used in combination with a cleansing agent and as an exfoliating tool, too.

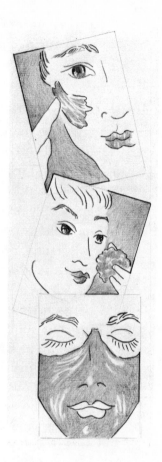

Exfoliation (Granular Scrub)

In addition to your soap or liquid cleanser, you should select a granular cleansing product to help slough off the dead skin cells which muddle together at the surface of the skin. (Brasivol and Pernox are examples of granular cleansing products.) There are many other scrubbing grains available that are suitable for oily or blemished skin. By using "grains" you'll scrape off the top layer of skin, leaving it smooth and glowing.

Toning

Following the granular scrub, you'll want to apply a toning solution. This step should serve to remove any remaining trace of make-up grime, while helping the skin look firm and smooth. If your skin is oily, you can select either a toning lotion, an alcohol-based astringent or a skin freshener. In shopping for the right toning product you should consider carefully its alcohol content. For very oily skin, a toner with a higher level of alcohol is suitable as alcohol serves as a drying agent. If your skin is less oily, choose a product with a lower alcohol content. Ten-O-Six Lotion by Bonnie Bell is an astringent for oily skin. Almay and Physicians Formula also have good astringents formulated for oily skin.

Moisturizing/Nourishing

As a woman moves into the 21-28 year cycle and beyond, the skin naturally becomes less oily. If you're over twenty-five and your skin is oily you still need to apply a moisturizer. The type of moisturizer and the amount of application depend on the oiliness of your skin. For a very oily complexion you should choose a light, nongreasy moisturizing lotion. A lotion of this type will be refreshing and will help retain a healthy supply of water in your skin. An example of such a product is Almay's Extra Light Night Cream. If you need a day cream as well, it should be a very light textured moisturizer.

By the time you've reached twenty-five or even before (depending on your skin's condition), you should realize the need for a pre-make-up or day cream to enable smoother application of make-up while moisturizing the skin during the day. For very oily skin, skip this step or use cream only in normal to dry spots. A throat cream to protect the neck area from exposure to the elements and prevent sagging; and an eye lubricant, which improves the skin's appearance in the eye area will also be needed. Finally apply a night cream before sleep. Usually, throat and night creams can be used interchangeably. However, you should select a lubricant (rather than a cream) for the protection of skin around your eyes and a pre-make-up cream that is compatible with your make-up foundation. In many cases, a regular cold cream or moisturizer will not allow even coverage of make-up foundation and thus is not effective as a pre-make-up cream. So, be sure to experiment a bit with the creams before stocking up. If your skin is oily, you can try a "moisturizing blotting lotion," instead of a regular facial moisturizer. However, your neck/throat area should still be given regular moisturizing treatments.

Stimulation _____

To promote the development of skin that is firm, smooth, and healthy-looking, you should become a consistent user of masques, which will be discussed in a later chapter. There are many wonderful types of masques, some of which can be made at home and most of which are inexpensive. The two most common types of masques are gel and clay. An oily skin can benefit from the alternative use of both types, although the gel is generally used to stimulate dry skin and the clay or mud type for oily skin. Examples of masques that you might use include Revlon's Skin Sluffing Almond Masque, Revlon's Deep Cleansing Clay Masque, Almay's Deep Pore Cleansing Masque, and Helena Rubenstein's Fresh Cover Brush on-Peel-off Masque.

CARING FOR DRY SKIN

Most women will begin to experience the first effects of dry skin during the twenties. Whether the skin starts to become dry sooner or later depends on how well you've cared for your face throughout the years. If you've practiced good nutrition, stayed away from too much sun, and adhered to a regular and effective cleansing routine, you have done your personal best in preventing the onset of dryness and will likely not be afflicted with truly dry skin during your twenties. But even if you've taken good care of your face, it will have been subjected to climatic and environmental elements which may encourage or delay the presence of dry, flaky skin. In addition, your parents' skin type is another factor contributing to your own skin's basic condition.

Make-up Removal and Cleansing _____

While a mild quality soap can be safely used on oily skin, it's a definite no-no for the dry-skinned. Soap tends to strip off not only dead cells on the skin's surface, but takes away the outer layer of oil, leaving the skin without its protective cover that prevents excessive loss of cellular moisture. Especially if your face is prone to dryness and you're in your late twenties or older, you should stay away from regular soap which includes virtually every type except for the special super-fatted lubricating soaps. Your best bet is to go for one of many excellent greaseless liquid cleaners.

Try choosing a washing cream with extra moisturizing agents if your face is very dry. For moderate to slightly dry skin, choose either a washing foam or cream cleanser or combine this method with occasional use of a special type of soap. Such "special" soaps include Purpose for Dry Skin, Keri Facial Soap, or Alpha Keri Moisturizing Bar. Examples of other appropriate cleansing agents for dry skin include Shiseido's Cleansing Foam, Elizabeth Arden's Fluffy Cleansing Cream, and Cetaphil Lotion Skin Cleanser. Whichever product you choose, don't forget to splash on some cool water to work your cleanser into a lather and remove as much as possible of the built-up surface residue. In selecting a cleanser you'll want to shop for one that thoroughly cleanses the face, without removing or otherwise disturbing the precious oil/water balance that is necessary for fighting the dry-skin battle.

Exfoliation (Granular Scrub) ───────────────────────────

Dry skin tends to become flaky, giving off a muddled and dull appearance and resulting in an extra accumulation of dead cells. To prevent this appearance, dry skin should be cleansed with a granular-type scrub (preferably an oil-based product to discourage further drying). For maximum effectiveness, gauge your granular cleansing treatments according to your own skin's special needs. The drier your skin is, the more often you'll need to apply this type of treatment. But be careful not to over-scrub and not so often that your skin becomes raw or irritated. With a little careful experimenting, you'll be able to schedule your exfoliating routine to suit your facial needs. An example of a granular scrubbing product suitable for dry skin is Cabot's Honey and Almond Scrub or Adrien Arpel's Honey and Almond Scrub. There are also many home-made dry skin scrubs that are effective and surely less expensive than commercially marketed products.

If your skin is especially sensitive, do stay away from harsh ingredients including highly fragranced products and those that contain large grains which may be too rough on your facial tissue. You may also use a product such as Buff-Puff or Buff-Puff for sensitive skin along with your soap-replacement cleanser. Again, go gentle on the scrubbing or your face may become red, patchy or irritated.

Toning

Toners are needed to stimulate and rejuvenate the facial skin and to improve its appearance. Dry skin, in particular, often becomes flaky and dull-looking and the use of toners can help greatly in tightening the pores while also smoothing and refreshing the skin. After a thorough cleansing, apply a very mild astringent or freshener. But be careful in your product selection. Most astringents on the market contain alcohol, a drying agent. If your skin is dry the last thing to do is apply an astringent with a high percentage of alcohol. Some products will claim to be alcohol-free but will contain other chemicals with the same drying power as alcohol. Therefore, you should read the labels, and if necessary, consult with a skin expert to insure that the product is, indeed, suitable for your skin type.

The use of a good astringent does have a very positive effect on the skin. Not only will the skin feel refreshed, but it will look firmer and wrinkles will be temporarily less noticeable. In general, astringents are more effective in tightening pores than are fresheners. However, if your skin is very dry, you should go with a skin freshener, rather than an astringent. Examples of dry skin toners include Shiseido's Facial Astringent Lotion Mild (low concentration of alcohol), Lancome's Tonique Douceur (non-alcoholic freshener), and Ten-O-Six Light by Bonne Bell (small amount of alcohol).

In addition to astringents and fresheners, other important facial toners include facial masques and facial saunas. These two steps can be very beneficial to any type of skin, but are absolute musts for dry skin, which need extra stimulation and nourishment to keep it smooth and glowing. Different types of masques and sauna treatments are discussed in Chapter 10.

Moisturizing/Nourishing

Once the toning routine is complete you should moisturize your skin. This step serves not only to restore some of the oils extracted while cleansing and toning, but it also aids the skin in retaining water. Before applying any moisturizer, dampen your skin with water. Then with the skin still slightly wet, proceed to moisturize. Applying moisturizing agents to a damp skin will serve to lock in water which is a moisturizing benefit you don't want to miss. Good moisturizers, applied properly, provide two major benefits to the skin: They reduce the level of dryness and assist the skin in retaining moisture (water). When a healthy supply of water is retained in the skin it stretches and is plumped up, which makes wrinkles and bags less noticeable. If you're in your late twenties or beyond, you should search for more than one good moisturizer. Among the products you should have in your facial wardrobe are:

Day Cream
Night Cream
Eye Cream
Throat Cream

- A good day cream consists of a pre-make-up base — a lightweight non-sticky, velvety cream that can be easily smoothed over the entire face. Shiseido's Pre-Make-Up Cream is a good example of such a product. Using a day cream under your make-up will allow it to go on much easier, resulting in an even, finished appearance.

- You can choose from among many excellent dry-skin night creams which will nourish your face as you rest. It's good not to interchange your day and night creams, except in the event where one cream serves both purposes equally well. Many regular night creams applied under make-up are too heavy or too greasy to be combined with a make-up foundation. If the two products are incompatible the foundation may not provide smooth coverage. Instead, your make-up can look spotty or may dissolve too readily into the cream, leaving either a greasy or muddled appearance, or both. On the other hand, day creams usually do not provide enough concentration to totally moisturize the face overnight. During these hours of rest, your face can use a more concentrated cream — a heavier moisturizer that will absorb slowly but provide greater penetration into the inner layers of your skin. So, be selective and choose different creams that match your skin's type and texture. Nutraderm is a lightweight cream designed for dry skin. It is also lanolin free which is helpful for skin that tends toward frequent breakouts. (Lanolin seems to encourage clogged pores and breakouts in some people.) For those who have few concerns with breakouts, Lubriderm (contains lanolin) can provide an effective moisturizing base. Purpose Dry Skin Cream (no lanolin) is a heavier moisturizer more appropriate as a night cream. Another example of a moisturizing product for normal to dry skin is Lancome's Hydrix Hydrating Creme. For dry to very dry skin, a night cream product such as Ultima II's Moisture Renewal Extra Rich Night Creme is suitable.

- Eye Cream — As women reach their late twenties (sometimes slightly before or after) small wrinkles and bags begin to appear under the eye area. To make this condition less noticeable, an eye cream lubricant is needed since a standard cream will not be effective in treating the eye area. A "lubricant" is necessary to plump up the skin, while making lines and traces less obvious. Although the effects of eye cream application are temporary, if one begins this treatment in the twenties and uses a good product consistently, the onset of wrinkles, bags and sags may be delayed considerably. And the skin in the eye area will certainly appear more firm and youthful looking than no treatment or if poor products were applied inconsistently. There are many eye creams available at a very moderate price. An example is Max Factor's Eye Cream Plus.

• For women who are concerned about keeping their neck attractive-looking, regular use of an appropriate throat cream should be part of the daily beauty routine. To "cream" this area, you may choose a special throat cream, a cold cream mixture, or even a night cream.

Stimulation

Regardless of your skin type, the consistent use of masques will rejuvenate and revitalize your skin. There are masques for virtually every kind of skin problem — from oily skin to dry, from blemished to sagging, lusterless or aged skin.

Dry skin can benefit greatly from the use of masques. After the masque is applied, it creates a protective shield which locks in water and penetrates deeply into the skin's tissue. Another benefit comes from the tightening sensation of the masque which promotes a healthy circulation in the skin. Then, as the masque is peeled or washed off, so are the dry flaky cells that have built upon the skin's surface. The result is skin that is much more smooth and lusterous.

You should use a gel-type masque if your skin is dry. These masques lock moisture into the skin and help combat flakiness, without stripping the skin's natural oils. Revlon's Moisturizing Honey Masque and Almay's Gentle Gel Masque are examples. Clay masques provide the same basic function as gel masques, but they may also rob the skin of its surface oils. Although beneficial for oily skin and even normal skin, they are not adviseable for the dry-skinned. In a later chapter, you will find examples of home-made masques that can be just as effective as commercially marketed ones.

The "masque" is one of the best dry-skin revivers, but there are other face-savers which are also quite helpful for dry skin. One such technique is the facial sauna. Spiced with an herb of your choice such as rose hips, peppermint, chamomile, or another, the sauna is an excellent means of treating dry skin. Not only does the sauna serve as a skin moisturizer, the steam penetrates and cleans the pores, allowing the accumulation of old make-up, creams, and pollution to be removed. Along with these pluses, the steam serves as a skin stimulator and promotes oil gland production as well.

❧ NORMAL SKIN CARE REGIMEN

It is rare to encounter a woman over thirty who believes her skin is "normal." So much has been said about the prevalence of dry skin that many women beginning in their twenties believe they are "victims" of dry skin, although this is not usually their true skin type. Since skin-type is affected by many diverse elements and can change quite rapidly, it's possible that skin can be normal at twenty-five and partially dry at 28-30. The factors involved in dryness are most often linked not only to biological aging and the genetic factor, but especially to eating and drinking habits, smoking, use of drugs, cosmetics containing drying agents, over-exposure to sun and intense climatic conditions, environmental substances, and other skin degenerators. Such factors contribute not only to dry skin but to an aged appearance. As far as normal skin goes, if you are still in your twenties and have not previously exposed your skin over long periods of time to the above-mentioned skin-killers, then you probably are not truly dry-skinned. Although you may experience a patch of dry skin now and then, this is not the characteristic which separates the dry-skinned from the normal. If you're thirty or older, the dry-skinned tendency increases, if for no other reason than the skin's natural aging process. Still, if your skin has been well cared for during the three decades hence, you probably are not yet a dry-skinned type.

Truly normal skin is actually very rare. In fact, most women have combination-type skin. Some parts are oily, some are dry and some in-between. However, if the skin's oil, moisture, and acid mantle are all balanced and there are no signs of dry or oily patches, the skin may be normal or "balanced."

Make-Up Removal and Cleansing

Normal skin should be cleansed by using a liquid or cream cleanser, an unscented, superfatted soap, or some combination of these two methods. Before cleansing, try applying a standard cold cream to your face, (such as Pond's or Arden's Fluffy Cleansing Cream) rub it in, and remove with damp cosmetic pads or soft cloth. Now that the top layer of make-up is loosened and partially removed, wet your face and cleanse as usual with a liquid cleanser or "special soap" to take off all the make-up and other residue which has accumulated. Cleanse morning and evening with cool water (not cold). If you prefer to use soap as part of your cleansing regimen, choose from products such as Basis, Alpha Keri, or Purpose.

Exfoliation (Granular Scrub)

The scrub is healthy for normal skin and should be used as needed to slough off the dead skin cells and to rejuvenate the facial skin. After sloughing splash cool water on the face and follow with a lightweight moisturizer. Suitable granular scrubbing products include Pernox, Brasivol, Adrien Arpel's Honey and Almond Scrub or Vegetable Peel-Off. Sponge products such as Buff-Puff should be used regularly with a cleansing agent.

Toning

For normal skin, choose a mild toner with a low concentration of alcohol. Astringents are stronger than fresheners so the latter may be the best choice for toning. Products such as Revlon's Moon Drops Moisturizing Skin Toner, Elizabeth Arden's Velva Smooth Lotion, and Helena Rubenstein's Skin Dew Moisturizing Freshener are examples of skin toners for normal skin.

Moisturizing/Nourishing

Normal skin should be moisturized by first wetting the face a bit. Before applying make-up, use a pre-make-up moisturizer and follow with application of your foundation. In the evening, pay attention to moisturizing under the eyes (eye lubricant), on the neck area, and apply moisturizer to the face before sleep. All-purpose moisturizing agents for normal skin include products such as Physicians Formula Moisturizer, Lubriderm, Nivea, Albolene, and Vasoline Dermatology Formula Cream.

Stimulation _____

Normal skin can be effectively treated with both clay and gel masques. Clay masques are helpful in extracting oil and pollution build-up on the face and in deep-cleansing the skin. On the other hand, gel masques are great for rejuvenating typically normal skin that has been exposed to excessive heat, cold, or other conditions that dried the face beyond its normal state. Stimulating masques such as those mentioned for dry and oily skin may also be used on normal skin. Other examples include Physicians Formula Beauty Buffers (to be mixed with a cleansing lotion or cream) and Queen Helene's Mint Julep Masque (also useful for oily or blemished skin.)

✣ COMBINATION SKIN CARE

Most women have skin that is sometimes dry in one area, oily in another, and perhaps normal in still other spots. Caring for this type of skin calls for "balanced" treatment. Again, the products you choose should depend on your age, the type of environment in which you live (extremely hot or cold), and your personal habits which affect your skin type. If your skin is also sensitive, you should stay away from harsh products that contain fragrances, additives, dyes, and other chemicals which may cause irritation to your skin.

The skin regimen for combination skin is the same as for other types:

- Make-up Removal and Cleansing
- Exfoliation or Granular Scrub
- Toning
- Moisturize/Nourish
- Stimulate

The key to effectively caring for combination skin (which is often considered as normal since most women have more oil in the T-Zone area, for example, and less in the cheek region) is the same as for any skin type. First, you must make an accurate assessment of your skin in order to know how to properly care for it. Evaluating your skin correctly is not difficult. However, at the time of assessment your skin should be sparkling clean and you should analyze it carefully, closely, and in direct daylight. If you are not sure as to how your skin should be classified, seek the opinion(s) of knowledgeable skin experts.

After your skin has been carefully analyzed, you should make it your business to analyze those cosmetic products and techniques that you feel will enhance your skin. Becoming acquainted with common cosmetic and chemical terminology and learning to read and understand cosmetic labels is also part of the process. Unless you become familiar with the basics of cosmetic preparations and their effects on skin, chances are you'll be selecting the wrong products, many of which may be harmful to your skin over the long run.

3. The Basic Tools and Techniques of Skin Care

Every woman, regardless of her skin type, should follow five basic steps to insure proper care to the outer skin. As discussed in Chapter 2, these include make-up removal and cleansing, exfoliation, toning, moisturizing, and stimulating.

❧ MAKE-UP REMOVAL AND CLEANSING

If you wear make-up, then you should pay special attention to removing every bit of it. Leaving old make-up on your skin will only increase your chances of developing a dull, muddled complexion. Over the long run, skimping on make-up removal will age your skin more rapidly and lead to the formation of certain skin problems in the process. Although make-up removal is part of the cleansing process, cleansing is also a bit more. Even without make-up skin must be cleansed to remove the outer layer of dead cells and other debris that continue to accumulate and pollute the skin. If the skin is not properly and consistently cleansed, at least twice a day, it will not only look dull and unhealthy, but will result in the clogging of pores and the development of pimples, whiteheads, and related skin breakouts.

Your choice of cleansing products should be based on your skin type, as mentioned in the previous chapter. Let's look at the most common skin cleansing tools, their advantages and disadvantages.

Soap

The oldest cleansing agent and still a very common one is soap. There are bar soaps (usually containing sodium salts) and liquid soaps (containing potassium salts in addition to fatty acids and other ingredients). Listed below are the most common soap types, their basic characteristics and uses.

Deodorant Soaps

These soaps are not for the face but are useful on the body to prevent odor. Although they are rich in bacteria-fighting chemicals and such chemicals can effectively remove dirt, debris, and odor from the body surface, they are far too harsh for the cleansing of delicate facial skin.

Detergent Soaps

Detergent soaps may be synthetic or natural, but regardless of the exact composition, most are produced from petroleum derivatives. They do not contain fatty acids and are not actually soaps at all. Some such detergent "soaps" may be used as a body cleanser, but this is not an appropriate facial cleansing agent. Again, the toxicity of detergent soaps (whether in the form of a bar or liquid body soap) depends, as in all soaps, on the alkaline content. Some detergent "soaps" may actually be less alkaline than many regular soaps.

Castile Soap

Named after the Spanish region where it originated, this soap is derived from olive oil and sodium hydroxide. It is usually white or egg shell in color and is basically equivalent to a standard toilet soap in its neutral effect on the body skin.

Acne Soap

Such soaps most often contain fine, medium, or coarse grains designed to slough off the dead skin cells and penetrate into clogged pores. Medications to prevent the spread of acne are also included in these products. Acne soap, because of its composition, can be drying and harsh, as well as irritating to some skin. It is best used under the supervision of a dermatologist for the treatment of acne or black-heads.

Transparent Soap

See-through or transparent soap is usually advertised as a dry skin product. However, alcohol and glycerin, added ingredients in this soap, tend to extract water from the skin. Although this soap is not appropriate for oily or acne skin (lack of ingredients to effectively remove oil), it is acceptable for normal skin. Neutrogena and Pears are good examples of transparent soaps.

French Milled Soaps

These soaps are designed low in alkaline and promoted primarily for dry skin. However, there are other soaps on the market with similar qualities and a less expensive price tag. Some of these soaps include Purpose, Keri, and Basis.

Superfatted Soaps

These soaps are designed with additional oils or fatty acids and as such, are supposed to serve as a moisturizing agent for dry skin. Because of their increased oil content, they are not as effective in removing all debris from the skin. However, since some oil remains on the skin's surface, the problem of dry skin is less likely to occur. In choosing a suitable superfatted soap, you should do a patch test first as some soaps are known to produce an allergic reaction, rash, or irritation to the skin. Superfatted soaps are milder than many, but to protect your skin from undue irritation, you should experiment a little before patronizing a particular brand.

There are various other soaps which are widely advertised but should not be used on the face. One such product is the "floating bar" which is a basic soap with extra water and air lodged inside. (Contains nothing of benefit to facial skin.) Another is cocoa-butter soap. In this one, cocoa butter (theobroma oil) is the primary fat ingredient. This cleansing bar is not advised for the face as it may cause allergic reactions. However, because of its softening and lubricating qualities, it is an excellent body soap. (Patch test first.) Some of the current fad soaps include those with fruit, vegetable, and herbal extracts. Although these soaps are attractively packaged and advertised, their natural essence is destroyed in the manufacturing process. Living plants quickly rot and before they can be used in cosmetics, they must be treated and preserved with various chemicals. In addition, fragrances are added to make them smell like a living fruit, vegetable, or herb. In general, the primary ingredients of these soaps include fats, salt, and water — the same essential ingredients found in basic soaps. Unless there are additional ingredients which may have a beneficial effect on skin, such soaps do not have any special skin care quality.

If you decide to cleanse your face with soap, be sure that your skin is wet before applying the soap. Then apply evenly over entire face and work up a lather. Rub gently and thoroughly around the face to rub off the dead cells and remove the built-up grime. To rinse, use warm or cool water (not cold, icy, or hot). Hot water opens the pores and releases water content within your skin. And while overly hot water can dehydrate the skin, icy water can irritate it. Don't forget to rinse carefully so that all soap is removed.

Other Cleansing Agents

Cleansing Creams and Lotions

These agents are promoted for their ability to loosen surface debris, to dissolve oil in the pores, and to quickly and thoroughly remove the build up of dirt. Although some dermatologists recommend this form of cleanser, many others will say that soap and water can do the job as effectively, with less chance of irritation. The choice is up to you and after experimenting with both soap and various creams/lotions, you will know which you prefer. Although soap is less expensive, some creams and lotions can remove debris more easily, while providing a moisturizing base to the skin. The most common types of cleansing creams are cold creams, liquefying cleansing creams, and washing creams.

Cold Creams

The basic cold cream formula includes beeswax, borax, mineral oil, and water. Today, however, there are many brands available with different chemical mixtures. When applied to the skin, the water-soluble ingredients in cold creams evaporate on the face and give off a cooling sensation. Hence, the name "cold" cream. The cream formula helps dissolve surface oils and loosen dead cells. Since cold cream residue does not come off with water alone, a tissue or soft towel is used to remove the cream. After removing the cream, it is good to rinse the face with warm water to get rid of any remaining residue.

Liquefying Creams

These creams are similar in composition to basic cold creams with the addition of other ingredients such as paraffin and petrolatum. This chemical mixture is formulated to melt on contact with the skin; the resulting oily film is supposed to be effective in dissolving clogged oils in the pores and in loosening dead cells and grime. Liquefying creams, like cold creams, must be removed with a tissue or towel and a final rinsing with water is again needed.

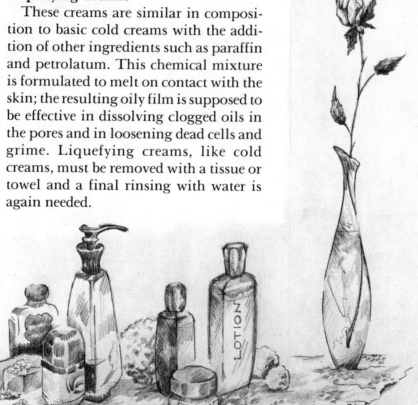

Washing Creams

These creams are a variation of liquefying creams, except that they are water soluble. This means that after application, they can be thoroughly rinsed off with warm water. Washing creams do provide a thorough cleansing and are easy on the sensitive facial skin.

Cleansing Lotions

This type of cleansing agent is available in liquid form and serves the same purpose as cleansing creams. The standard mixture for cleansing lotions contains mineral oil, triethanolamine stearate, and water.

Selecting a Cleansing Agent

The American Medical Association and many dermatologists say that soap and water do as well as creams/lotions, are cheaper and provide less chance for irritation or allergy. Nevertheless creams are good choices for normal and dry skin because of the oil they deposit on the skin, while soaps can cause drying. Creams, however, are not effective in cleansing oily skin.

Exfoliation

Exfoliation is another word for sloughing. The process involves removing outer layers of dead cells and is beneficial for all skin types. It cleans oily skin well and through scraping, helps open up clogged pores that may cause pimples and other breakouts. As strange as it may seem, the process of exfoliation is also excellent for dry skin. Instead of creating dryness, rubbing and scraping will remove dead cells that cause the dry and flaky skin. Not only will these dead cells be exfoliated, your skin will appear more smooth, glowing and healthy. In fact, one of the benefits of the exfoliation technique is that skin cells appear plumper and this plumpness causes fine lines and wrinkles to become temporarily less noticeable. Remember, this effect is temporary, which is why it's important to include exfoliation in your daily skin care regimen. With regular exfoliation, the skin looks clearer and healthier because dead skin cells are removed and new skin growth is stimulaged.

Normal and combination skin also look better with regular exfoliation because the dead cells are consistently removed and blood circulation is improved, giving off the glowing appearance that women so often seek.

Before exfoliating your facial skin, you must first choose the proper cleansing products and the exfoliating tool. The products and tools you choose, as well as the frequency of exfoliation, should depend on your skin type and condition. While all skin types can benefit from this process, you don't want to overdo it by rubbing too hard or too long or exfoliating too often. You should base your decision about these things on common sense. Practice exfoliation in moderation as your skin adjusts to the process. If you can see any irritation, you're rubbing too hard and probably too long in one place.

Should you have any concerns, check with your dermatologist or skin care consultant. But do not be surprised if your dermatologist tells you that exfoliation is not that necessary or that you only need to scrub once a week. As in all professions, there are differences of opinion as to which methods and how much are beneficial. However, exfoliating or sloughing off dead cells can have only a positive effect on your skin if it is done with the proper products and tools and according to your skin's needs.

Basic exfoliation tools include washcloths, sponges, soft brushes, special pads such as buff puffs, and skin machines. Keep in mind that exfoliation is good not only for the face but for other areas of the body including the back and shoulders, neck, legs, and buttocks. If you do select a pad, sponge, soft brush, or washcloth, be sure to have one for the face and another for the body. Skin machines with soft rotating brushes can be used to exfoliate but specially designed pads or brushes are just as good. Some people prefer using only a washcloth. Unless your skin is extremely sensitive you will find that the pads, sponges, or brushes do a better job.

In the beginning you can scrub carefully for about a minute. If your tool is especially abrasive, (some pads and brushes are more abrasive than others) you should time yourself so that you don't overscrub. After your skin adjusts to this process, you can increase the time to two and then three minutes. Use a circular motion to scrub various areas. Remember, in problem areas it's best to scrub a little longer, but not harder. The best time to exfoliate is in the morning so that your skin will look its healthy best for the day. You can also scrub again in the evening if your skin needs the additional treatment.

Regardless of your skin type and the products and tools you use to exfoliate, you must follow with a rinsing routine. Splash several times with warm water and pat dry. If your skin is oily, you can apply an astringent to remove the final traces of residue from the skin. Those with dry skin can apply to slightly damp skin, a water-retaining moisturizer to keep the skin soft. More on moisturizers later.

Toning

Toning is the next step and is important to tighten your pores, wake up your skin a bit and to make fine lines and wrinkles temporarily less noticeable. All skin types need toning and to accomplish this effect, there are various types of toning lotions. These include astringents, fresheners, and clarifying lotions.

Astringent

This type of toning agent contains mostly alcohol with small amounts of boric acid, alum, menthol and other ingredients. When applied to the face astringents make the skin feel refreshed and tightened. It is often difficult to locate a suitable astringent since there are endless varieties, many of which are listed under other names such as pore lotions, refining lotions, toning lotion, and toners. A true astringent makes pores appear temporarily smaller and is effective for oily skin.

Because astringents contain alcohol and other drying agents, they are not to be used on dry skin. For normal and dry skin the best choice is a freshener which may contain only a tiny amount of alcohol or none at all. If your skin is oily you can experiment with various astringents until you find one that works well on your skin. For skin that is part oily and part normal to dry, you can also select a freshener and add ¾ teaspoon of alum (aluminum salt) to about 10 oz. of freshener. Witch hazel extract can serve as an astringent for normal to oily skin and when diluted with water may be applied as a toner for dry skin. Astringents are also recommended for acne. But again, the key is selecting a good product. You might ask your pharmacist or dermatologist to suggest a good one for your skin type and condition.

Fresheners

Although fresheners may contain some alcohol and other drying agents, the formula is much weaker than for astringents. Fresheners may contain bay rum, boric acid, chamomile, glycerin, menthol, lavender oil, aluminum salt, various herbal extracts, and other ingredients. Designed to make the skin feel cool, tightened, and refreshed, this is the toning lotion of choice for dry to normal skin. They may also be listed under skin tonics or freshening lotions.

Clarifying Lotions

Another type of toner, this one is promoted to make the skin clearer and smoother by removing the outer layer of dead cells and grime. These lotions usually contain water, glycerin, alcohol and a chemical that will break down keratin. (The substance that comprises much of the skin's outer layer.) Such chemicals may include salicylic acid, resorcinol and benzyl peroxide. According to law, these agents must be listed on the label. There are, however, other keratolytic agents that do not have to be listed on the product label.

Clarifying lotions may contain a high concentration of alcohol and may be highly alkaline as well. If you regularly exfoliate via the method earlier described, and have found a suitable astringent or freshener, there should be no real need for a clarifying lotion. However, if you are interested in experimenting, be sure to select a clarifying lotion with the contents listed on the label.

Moisturizing

Skin moisturizers are also referred to as emollients. These products may have many names and come in various forms. There are hand and neck creams, eye creams, skin nourishing creams, day creams, night creams, skin softeners, collagen creams, sprays, lotions and other products that fall under the listing of moisturizer. The purpose of a good moisturizer is to soften the skin to help fight dryness, irritation and cracking. In essence, a facial moisturizer should lock in the skin's own natural moisturizer, which is water. Moisturizers applied to the skin may "cover up" flakiness or dryness and the oil will help seal water into the skin. Skin is softened primarily by the water that's locked into the inner skin.

Whether you select a cream, lotion, or spray makes little difference to the skin. In fact, this choice is a matter of personal preference. All skin types can benefit from moisturizers but the quality and suitability of the product is important. When it comes to moisturizers and many other cosmetic products as well, price is not an indicator of quality. Most moisturizers contain the same basic ingredients including mineral oil, beeswax, lanolin, sorbitol, stearic acid and polysorbates. Higher priced products usually contain the basic emollient ingredients in addition to selected oils such as peanut, corn, almond, apricot, coconut, or some other oil. They are promoted as containing a "special" oil that will leave your skin softer. But there is little evidence to suggest that any one of these oils is better than the other. Ingredients such as emulsifiers, preservatives, antioxidants, antibacterials, and perfumes are also found in basic emollients.

Most women need only two moisturizers — one especially for day and one for night. Regular moisturizers are lighter than night creams which tend to be thicker and oilier.

Your choice of the right combination of moisturizers should depend on your skin type and what works best for you. While there are guidelines based on skin types, every skin is different. For example, if your skin is oily you should choose a moisturizer with light-weight oils and soothing agents and use it sparingly. Refer back to Chapter 2 for information on moisturizers and skin type.

Stimulating

There are two basic stimulating techniques: masques and saunas. Regardless of skin type or condition, regular application of a masque will provide an extra beauty boost for your complexion. Saunas are also helpful in loosening dead skin cells, in dissolving clogged oil in the pores, in stimulating circulation, and in providing extra moisture for the skin. You may purchase an electric facial sauna, utilize the sauna at your health club, or create a similar effect with a pot of hot water and a towel. More on this technique later.

Masques

Masques are used to perk up, stimulate and firm the skin, to temporarily tighten the pores and plump up wrinkles. Masques will not remove wrinkles or shrink pores, although some products may claim to do so.

There are two basic masque categories — gel and clay (often referred to as mud). As discussed in a later chapter, gel masques are best for dry skin and clay masques for oily. A masque, once removed, will make the skin feel refreshed and tightened.

As with toners, masques produce a slight irritation that tighten the pores and plumps up the skin around the wrinkles, making fine lines and wrinkles temporarily less noticeable. With a good masque, the end result is a complexion that is rosy, smooth, and glowing. Clay masques can serve as deep cleansing agents as they draw out oil and grime. On the other hand, gel masques help seal in moisture and restore water to normal or dry skin.

Both types of masques are spread over the entire face (avoiding the delicate skin around the eye area). After a specified time, the masque is peeled or washed off and with it goes the dead skin cells and debris that has built up and muddled the complexion. Masques often contain other ingredients such as herbal, fruit, and vegetable extracts. Some additives do benefit the skin temporarily and others do not. To find out which ones are effective, you should keep a glossary of cosmetic ingredients nearby and experiment to find out which ingredients suit your skin.

✤ TAKING TIME TO CARE FOR BODY SKIN

Body skin also needs its share of attention in order to appear healthy. The techniques are basically the same as for facial skin care, although the tools (products) are different.

Cleansing ——————————————————————————

This step is obvious enough and does not need much explanation. A mild body soap that is compatible with the needs of your skin will serve the purpose. You may choose a bar or liquid but it should not be a harsh soap, nor should it be a heavily fragranced one. Not only would a strong soap product be unsuitable for your body skin it would likely cause irritation to your delicate female parts.

Exfoliation, Toning, and Stimulation ——————————————————

Removing dead skin cells from the skin's top surface is just as important to healthy body skin as it is for the face. If you shave your legs three to four times a week then you are already taking off many of the dry, dead cells that build up on the outer layer. The best way to exfoliate other areas of the body is to use a body brush, a loofah, or special sponge with enough roughness to do the job. This process of scraping off body debris can be done every day in the bath or shower or only a few times a week as needed. In practicing this technique regularly you are also toning and stimulating the body skin. Additional skin toning and stimulation may occur by applying an oil such as mustard oil via massage to the entire body before showering.

This oil improves the skin tone, leaving it more lustrous than before. There are many other oils which may give similar results and you can experiment with them to see how your skin responds.

In addition to pre-shower oil application and massage, you can add bath oil to your bath to soften and tone the skin. The oils may come in the form of beads, in a box, or jar. They usually contain a small amount of alcohol, perfumed oil, soap and water. For dry skin, oils are especially recommended. Bubble baths are also used, but not to tone or soften the skin. Rather, the bubbles create a delightfully pleasant atmosphere and have a soothing effect. Bubble bath products with detergents should be selected carefully and used sparingly as they may irritate the vaginal area.

Moisturizing

Body skin, like facial skin, needs moisturizing to seal in water content and soften and smooth the outer layer. To moisturize body skin, you can select an all-purpose body lotion or cream as described in the facial care section. The best time to moisturize is immediately after showering or bathing while the skin is still slightly damp. However, you may apply body moisturizers at other times as well.

Along with moisturizers, the body skin also responds to bath powders (applied after a bath to soak up excess moisture), and anti-perspirants and deodorants. Anti-perspirants are composed of water, aluminum salts, and other ingredients similar to those in astringents. Aluminum salts make the skin around the sweat glands swell up in the pores and perspiration from the sweat ducts is retarded.

Deodorants do not inhibit the flow of perspiration but aid in controlling or eliminating bacterial growth on the skin. There are various kinds of deodorants including products containing chemicals that wipe out bacteria, products that destroy bacteria and control future growth, and deodorants that do not kill bacteria, but merely inhibit them from reacting with the perspiration to form odor.

Areas Requiring Special Attention _____

There are certain areas of the skin that tend to be more sensitive and more prone to aging: hands, upper chest, neck, and around the eyes. To minimize the impact of wear and tear, special attention should be given to these areas.

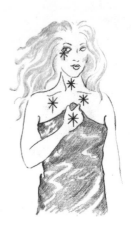

- **Hands** are constantly exposed and it's no wonder they should need extra care. The backs of hands, in particular, are prone to age and should be protected, whenever possible. For daytime care, it's a good idea to carry a hand lotion and use it periodically. Re-apply the moisturizer after washing hands; during the winter, hands should be creamed more often. For night care, apply a heavy cream to the hands and cover with cotton gloves for an all-night moisturizing routine. When you plan to be in the sun, remember to apply sunscreen. And for household chores and other tasks involving contact with harsh chemicals and cleansers, be sure to wear gloves.

- **Upper chest.** Young women often are unaware of the damage sun can do to this part of the skin. Since the upper chest is particularly sensitive, even moderate sun exposure can cause the early appearance of fine lines and loose skin.

  Usually, sun damage that occurs on the upper chest during the first twenty years will begin to show up in one's twenties and thirties. If additional damage occurs, the skin will age even more rapidly. This area should be moisturized every night with a concentrated body care lotion. A neck cream may also be used, depending on the condition of the skin. Again, this area needs extra special care while in the sun — a heavy sunscreen and limited exposure.

  For both the hands and upper chest, the five skin care steps apply and in the same order as discussed earlier. Step #2 (exfoliation) and Step #5 (stimulation) may be done on a weekly, rather than daily basis.

- **Neck.** Many women, especially young women in their twenties and thirties, pay little, if any attention, to the skin on the neck. Since skin in this area is also exposed to the elements and is not connected to muscle, it is especially prone to sagging and fine lines. Sun exposure, will of course, increase the aged-looking appearance.

  Early preventive skin care will provide good insurance against an aging neck. A bit of cream applied during the day and a full cream treatment every night is appropriate. There are many neck creams on the market that are rich in emollients. Use your good judgment and remember that price does not necessarily equal quality. An example of a neck creme is Estée Lauder's Swiss Neck Creme.

- **Eyes.** As discussed in Chapter 2, the skin below the eyes on the eyelid is vulnerable to bags and fine lines. This skin is very delicate and needs to be creamed lightly during the day. Before bedtime an eye lubricant (gel type substance), should be applied around the eye area. To decrease the appearance of fine lines or sagging skin under the eyes, a concealer to match your make-up foundation should be applied sparingly below the eye, around the corners, and on the eyelid. The forehead skin between the eyes is one more spot where lines tend to develop early on. One of the worst contributors to forehead lines is squinting and frowning. A good preventive measure is to go easy on squinting, keep current on your eye prescription (if you need glasses or contacts), and wear sunglasses whenever you are outdoors. Another reminder: Take care when applying and removing eye make-up as the inner and outer eye area can be irritated by certain chemicals found in cosmetic products.

4. The Impact of Lifestyle on your Skin

Developing and maintaining beautiful skin is a special kind of achievement that results not by accident, but through proper and consistent care and long-term protection from severe "skin-killers." As one advances in age, the skin's susceptibility to wrinkles, and other outward manifestations of aging naturally increase. Aging, however, is not the only factor involved in the onset of various skin disorders.

Along with physiological aging are other elements that promote skin deterioration, including the development of wrinkles. Each of these factors is discussed only briefly since their effects on general health are widely known. For very specific information regarding the impact of any one of these factors on the skin's health, you should refer to medical periodicals and reports in the fields of Dermatology, Nutrition and General Skin Care.

Abuse and Dehydration

Excessive exposure to sun, wind, cold, and other intense climatic conditions impair the skin and contribute to premature wrinkle formation. Severe skin dehydration and illness may also set the stage for an early onset of wrinkles.

Smoking

It has been established that smokers develop more wrinkles than do non-smokers. Smoking appears to impede blood circulation, which in turn results in food and oxygen being prevented from reaching the skin. At the same time, carbon monoxide and water accumulate within the cells and produce a polluted environment which facilitates wrinkle development. Smoking may ultimately impair the collagen structure, which is largely responsible for youthful-looking skin, and also depletes the body's supply of vitamin C an important vitamin for healthy collagen.

Heavy Drinking

Alcohol is known to be a drying agent and when consumed excessively, will tend to age skin much more rapidly than if abstinence or extreme moderation were practiced. Alcohol not only soaks up water and dehydrates tissues, it also hinders the metabolism of vitamins and robs the skin of valuable nutrients.

Facial Expressions

Wrinkle formation is encouraged when one consistently assumes an exaggerated expression such as squinting or frowning. Any expression that manipulates the skin deeply and consistently will ultimately leave its mark in the form of a wrinkle. Relaxation and moisturizing can help counteract these effects.

Natural Aging

As you advance in years, underlying tissues shrink and the skin becomes less elastic. Collagen production also slows down, causing the skin to become loose, lined, and wrinkled. To delay the effects of biological aging, you should be aware of the many skin killers mentioned in this chapter. And drinking plenty of water is recommended to help the skin retain moisture. Certain dermatological treatments, as discussed in Chapter 8, can be effective in improving the appearance of aged skin.

Too Much Massaging

Excessive rubbing of creams into the skin can contribute to the breakage of collagen fibers and the development of fine lines and wrinkles.

Taking precautions to guard against premature wrinkling is one form of skin care protection. Clearing the skin of pollution build-up, whiteheads, blackheads, and other skin problems can be a long and confusing process. But if you understand how personal habits, lifestyle, and environmental factors leave their mark on your face, then your success in developing and maintaining clearer skin will be greater.

❧ OTHER FACTORS AFFECTING THE SKIN'S CONDITION

In some cases, the facial skin may clear with proper care after adolescence. More often, however, women experience periodic break-outs throughout a large part of their lives. Many adult skin break-outs are related to personal and environmental factors that can be managed to enable healthier looking skin. Such factors include:

- Cosmetics
- Drugs
- Menstrual Cycle
- Sun
- Stress
- Diet
- Environmental Elements
- Pregnancy
- Genetics

Cosmetics

Choosing the wrong products — those that are unsuitable for your skin type — can lead to skin irritation and breakouts. By becoming familiar with cosmetic terminology and learning to rec-ognize the chemical culprits that wreak havoc with your skin, you'll save your face from a lot of unneccessary disturbances.

Drugs

It's impossible to pinpoint exactly which drugs may cause skin eruptions because individual reactions to drugs vary greatly. Certain drugs, however, are known widely for their negative effects on skin. Some of these include: lithium, dilantin, danazol, danocrine, and steroids in all forms. The birth-control pill has a positive effect on the skin of some women and a very negative impact on the skin of others. A common sense approach to the drug issue is to do without, unless the drug is indispensible to your health and harmless to your skin.

Menstrual Cycle

Usually, the periodic breakout, if a woman is prone to it, will occur about a week before the cycle is to begin. Apparently responsible for these cyclical eruptions are three hormones involved in the menstrual process — progesterone, estrogen, and testosterone. The testosterone hormone is usually cited as a factor in skin eruptions but during the menstrual cycle, an increase in the progesterone level also contributes to skin flare-ups. As the progesterone levels decrease prior to the onset of the cycle, it is thought that the eruptions begin to subside. To cope with the skin aggravations induced by the menstrual cycle, forget trying to manipulate hormones and focus more closely on your daily cleansing and skin care regimen.

Sun

Excessive exposure to sun not only causes long-term damage to the skin, but may also, in some persons, cause short-term or immediate skin flare-ups. As with smoking, ultraviolet radiation damages the collagen structure and promotes the early appearance of aged skin. Sunlight abuse can also harm the blood vessels of the dermal layer, which supply vital nutrients and oxygen to the skin. Your best approach is to keep your face well protected and avoid prolonged exposure to the sun. Another word of warning is to stay out of the sun while on medications. Certain medications combined with sun may cause skin rashes and breakouts in some persons, if not a more serious bodily reaction.

Prolonged Stress

This factor is a major contributor to facial breakouts. Although all other factors may be under control, chronic, destructive stress that becomes a routine part of daily life can blotch up even the most well-kept face. Stress can promote pimples almost immediately if the body's resistance is already low. Or in a delayed fashion, a stressful situation can stimulate adrenal glands to step up production of hormones. Generally, the pimples will follow anywhere from 10 days to a month after a major stressful encounter. Since everyone experiences stress, the key is to minimize "destructive" stress situations. Temporary, constructive stress can be very uplifting and may even have a positive effect on the skin.

Diet

Nutrition, in relation to skin health, is certainly a personal, and also environmental factor in the sense that each person is responsible for selecting her nutritional menu from the larger environment. Unfortunately, many foods are contaminated or polluted with chemicals that may cause allergies, skin reactions, and even more serious health problems over the long run. The topic of food contamination is beyond the scope of this book, but it is surely an area to keep current on as new information becomes available. The nutritional aspects of skin care are discussed in the next chapter.

Environmental Pollutants

The many sources of environmental pollution and their possible relation to skin problems are far too numerous to name. Chemical skin-killers may be found in the form of fumes in the workplace, in the home, in open air and water, and even in some foods. Keep your eyes open for chemically infested atmospheres and avoid contact when possible. Finally, keep hands away from your face except when cleansing and applying make-up. Keep in mind that central heating and air conditioning deplete moisture from the skin, as will a hot and dry climate.

Pregnancy

Pregnancy is known to encourage skin breakouts, especially during the first three months. This is the time when estrogen and progesterone hormones are in a state of flux, and their constant fluctuating wreaks havoc on the skin. After the first three months, however, estrogen levels rise and the skin usually clears up. (As estrogen levels increase, oil production is decreased and the skin becomes less susceptible to breakouts.)

Additional skin problems may be experienced after birth as estrogen levels drop down again. Be prepared by keeping other skin factors under control and especially stick to a well-designed skin care regimen.

Genetic Predisposition

Although the above-mentioned factors affecting skin health are within personal control, you obviously cannot erase the hereditary blueprint which influences your skin's appearance and its changes through the years. What you can do is understand the genetic pattern in regard to your skin and then treat it appropriately. Look at your skin's texture and color and notice your parents' skin. Certainly, you cannot make hard and fast assumptions about your skin's future just by checking out your parents' skin, as their habits, circumstances, and exposure to the elements will have been different from yours. But you should take into consideration the basic characteristics of skin type, texture, and color. For example, you should realize that dry-skinned complexions are more likely to develop tiny surface lines than oily or normal skin types. Dry skin is thought to be thinner than oily skin and more sensitive to internal and structural changes. Very dry and pale complexions are also prone toward broken capillaries and other skin discolorations.

5. Feeding your Skin Nutritionally

The science of nutrition is still in its infancy. A lot is known but there is a lot more to be discovered. What is known, however is often ignored, taken for granted, or considered boring, because of our established lifestyle patterns. To many of us, the thought of a "diet" or dietary control is particularly unpleasant. Immediately, we think of eating bland, tasteless food or even skipping meals entirely. Of course, such erroneous conceptions take their toll on our bodies —both inside and out.

While poor nutritional patterns impair internal organs over the long run, the impact on our skin is much more immediate. Since the skin is the most exposed of all bodily organs, it is constantly in contact with destructive pollutants — from harsh cosmetic preparations to sun, wind, heat, and a myriad of chemicals in our home, work, and leisure environments. With this kind of intense external exposure, the skin is already fighting an uphill battle. When external factors are combined with internal bodily pollution such as inadequate nutrition habits, smoking, and consumption of drugs and alcohol, the skin becomes a vulnerable, if not extremely fragile organ which must be carefully protected in order to be preserved.

Proper nutritional practice involves not just perseverance or will power but a whole lot of applied common sense. Whether you're trying to lose or gain weight, or maintain the status quo, the key is to eat intelligently. For good skin and good health that means no extreme overeating or undereating and reprogramming dietary behavior, if necessary, to maintain a balanced nutritional program. To be sure, there is no one way to diet, nor any ideal diet. One of the worst things that skin can be subjected to is a series of rapid and frequent weight gains and losses. Not only is erratic dieting unhealthy for the body as a whole, it has an aging effect on the skin, leaving it loose and sagging. When dieting to lose or gain weight is necessary, it should be carried out intelligently, preferably under the advice of a trusted physician or nutritionist/dietician. And whatever the specific dietary plan may include, the dieting process itself should take place at a reasonable pace. (One to two pounds a week is considered safe and reasonable).

A serious attempt to alter one's nutritional patterns requires not only changes in poor eating habits, but also changes in basic lifestyle, shopping, food preparation and meal scheduling practices. It is essential to throw out old habits that are detrimental to nutritional progress.

One of the most important aspects of nutrition for both weight, health, and skin care maintenance what Dr. Roger Williams calls "biochemical individuality."* He reminds us that to diet successfully, we have to remember that we are each individual and unique, with different dietary needs. Consequently, individual dietary requirements may deviate greatly from any published diet plan.

As nutritionist Carlton Fredericks once noted, any "printed" diet plan is wrong — a diet must be created for an individual, not for the news media. The bottom line regarding "diets" is to experiment and adopt those patterns (eating, lifestyle, etc.) that allow you most control over food, your weight, and appearance. It is equally important to learn to "flex" such patterns to accommodate changes in health, social, and personal matters. Food can and should be one of the pleasures of life. Too often it ends up abused or a source of pain.

---

* Roger J. Williams, *Nutrition Against Disease* (New York: Pitman Publishing Corp., 1971). Also R. J. Williams, *Biochemical Individuality* (New York: Wiley, 1963).

❧ PRESERVING YOUR SKIN THROUGH INTELLIGENT FOOD SELECTION

For good health in general and healthy skin in particular, eating intelligently means knowing which foods to pass up or take in moderation and which to include regularly in your diet. For example, excessive consumption of sugar is one of the typical pitfalls. We are all aware that soda, candy, cakes, and pastries contain sugar, but so many other products contain refined sugar as well. White flour products, coca-cola, and certain canned fruits and breakfast cereals are packed with sugar. Check the labels of food products and become attuned to how much sugar you are actually consuming. Most of us know which foods fall into the "junk food" category. But as a reminder, we should consume in moderation those foods heavy in starch and sugar including white bread, ice cream, pasta, and the like. Such foods contribute virtually nothing to building, repairing, and maintaining body tissues. They add nothing in the form of valuable nutrients and once consumed are easily converted to fat. Furthermore, "junk foods" are the demons most often responsible for skin problems. Indulging in these foods does not even satisfy the hunger urge, leaving you as hungry as before the binge.

What happens is that refined sugars and starches are digested and absorbed within the blood stream very quickly. This digestion process rapidly breaks sugars and starches into glucose — one of the body's prime energy sources — but the body needs to develop its store of glucose more slowly from foods which are slowly converted into glucose and filtered into the blood. Like alcohol and caffeine, consuming sugar in the form of junk food can become addictive — having the same impact on the blood sugar level.

Sugar is an important ingredient for all of the body's cells as an ultimate energizer. But the form in which you consume sugar is the crucial factor. The safest way to satisfy the body's sugar requirement is to combine natural foods consisting of carbohydrates such as whole grains, fruits and vegetables; dairy products; proteins such as fish, eggs and meat; and fat sources such as nuts, avocados, and cheese. These foods allow sugar to be filtered slowly into the blood while also insuring that a high level of energy is maintained. In keeping your blood sugar level high, the desire for sweets and sudden energy boosts practically disappear.

Processed foods provide additional health-related risks. The main trouble with such foods is that they contain little nutritional value. Usually, the nutritious elements have been removed or they have been sprinkled with additives that may prove harmful to health —particularly in the long run. Some of the foods which fall into this category are frozen dinners, canned foods, sausages, white rice, sugared cereals, french fries, hot dogs, and white flour. Additives are used in food to give color, flavor, or longer shelf life. There are flavorings, preservatives, colorings, stabilizers, emulsifiers, and antioxidants found in food for various reasons. For example, coloring can be found in many candies, weiners, cheeses, and sweet potatoes. Emulsifiers are used by bread manufacturers to make bread softer, so that it looks fresher and has a longer shelf life. Between the emulsifier and the white flour content, there is not much of value in white bread. Then there are synthetic antioxidants to aid in preventing spoilage of refined oils and fats. These are made from petroleum products and added to bacon, butter, shortening, potato chips, doughnuts, cake, pastries, candies, cookies, peanut butter, and candied fruit, to name a few. It is thought that synthetic antioxidants can cause allergies, skin problems and breathing problems and perhaps more serious health problems with long-term exposure. The list of chemicals used in food processing and preservation is long and beyond the scope of this chapter.

Additional poisons to be found in some foods include chemicals entering the food as residues of pesticides, fertilizers, environmental pollutants, and cattle feeds.

The U.S. Senate Select Committee on Nutrition and Human Needs concluded after extensive studies, testimony, and investigations, the importance of the nutrition concern:

> "We have reached the point where nutrition or the lack or excess or the quality of it, may be the nation's number one public health problem. The threat is not beri-beri, pellagra, or scurvy. Rather we face the more subtle, but also more deadly, reality of millions of Americans loading their stomachs with foods which is likely to make them obese, to give them high blood pressure, to induce heart disease, diabetes, and cancer — in short, to kill them over the long term."*

If nutrition abuse is powerful enough to impair our internal organs, we can be certain that our skin, the most exposed and delicate of all bodily organs, is also greatly affected by faulty nutrition and poor eating habits.

❧ THE EFFECT OF FOOD ELEMENTS ON SKIN

Foods such as chocolate, french fries and other greasy foods are no longer considered a major cause of acne. But these and other foods do tend to aggravate skin disorders in some people. If you are prone to skin disorders and feel that a certain food has contributed to your condition, you should reduce or eliminate it from your diet, regardless of what current research now indicates. If the food is a dietary essential (such as milk products) you may try reducing your intake or find an appropriate substitute.

Although the above foods are not known to affect hormones, there are some food and drug substances that do appear to affect or influence hormones and their stimulation of the oil glands. These include iodides, bromides, and androgen.

Iodide (or iodine), found in food and drugs, is known to increase skin breakouts, especially in people who are acne-prone. After iodide

---

* U.S. Senate (Select Committee on Nutrition and Human Needs), "Nutrition and Health: An Evaluation of Nutritional Surveillance in the United States" (Washington, D.C.: Government Printing Office, 1975), p. 5.

filters into the bloodstream, excess is eliminated by way of the oil glands. During this process of elimination, iodide aggravates the pores and causes skin breakouts. To control your intake of iodide, you should be aware of certain food elements which contain aggravating levels of this substance. Such foods include, but are not limited to the following:

- *Liver and kidney meat*
- *Junk foods* containing high levels of salt. (e.g. tortilla and potato chips)
- *Iodized salt*
- *Some seafood that is high in protein. Kelp,* in particular, contains very high levels of iodide. Some of the most popular seafood such as sole, red snapper, oysters, and shrimp have been found to contain relatively low levels of iodide.
- *Peanuts*
- *Vitamin and mineral supplements* may contain iodide and kelp.
- *Milk.* High levels of iodide have been found in some milk products. As with meat, the source of iodide has been linked to cowlick salt.
- *Asparagus, broccoli, wheat germ,* and *white onions* also contain relatively high levels of iodide.

Iodide may be found in other foods and other sources. Skin flare-ups in those who are susceptible may occur when large quantities are consumed as well as when iodide comes in contact with the skin. Consuming a particular food high in iodide may not induce a skin problem, but ingesting large quantities through various foods and sources may worsen acne in susceptible people.

Bromide is similar to iodide in the effect it has on acne. It is found in many cold medications and other drugs. Since drug manufacturers are not required to list every ingredient on the product label, it may not be listed as an ingredient. Your pharmacist can usually clarify any concern regarding ingredients.

The concern with androgen is primarily linked to certain birth control pills. Androgen refers to all male hormones — testosterone, in particular. Some birth control pills, especially many of the "mini pills," fall into the androgen-oriented category. These pills, which are high in androgens, stimulate oil production in some women and cause acne to worsen. Some of the androgen-oriented pills include Lo-Ovral, Ovral, and Norinyl. Although these mini pills are considered safer with fewer side effects such as blood clots and migraines — they have been linked to acne flare-ups.

On the other hand, estrogen-oriented pills such as Demulen, Enovid, and even Orthonovum have been known to clear up acne in many cases. Ingesting the synthetic estrogen causes hormone production in the ovaries to stop. The estrogen influx thus lowers the production of testosterone in the ovaries, (About fifty percent of a woman's testosterone is developed in the ovaries.) less oil is produced by the oil glands and acne conditions improve.

In general, androgen-oriented pills worsen skin problems and estrogen-oriented pills improve the condition. However, research has also shown an identical pill to have different effects on different women. Therefore, individual reactions to the same pill can vary greatly. In essence, the effects of ingesting synthetic hormones can be complicated and the choice of which pill, if any, is a personal one.

Generally, foods or drugs containing these substances should be consumed in small amounts by people who are susceptible to a reaction. Eating a few cashews, for example, should not cause skin problems. But eating an entire bag of nuts may activate a skin breakout. Some people report allergic reactions to other foods as well. But individuals vary in their reactions to foods and medications and if you do feel that a particular food is disturbing your skin, you should avoid it and seek professional guidance, if necessary.

As mentioned before, excessive and/or frequent consumption of very hot and spicy foods, along with heavy consumption of caffeine and alcohol can cause an enlargement of blood vessels in the skin (vasodilation). The result is the unattractive appearance of small red lines on the face or other areas of the body.

❧ WHY EAT

We normally eat out of hunger and for pleasure. If we eat slowly, our appetite is satisfied with less food. If we chew the food, we aid the digestive process. If not, we often disrupt the digestive tract, take in more food than we should, and lose the pleasure of eating altogether. The best way, then, is to chew your food well. If you've not already developed this habit, you'll find that in chewing slowly your blood sugar level starts to rise. When it does rise, it relays a message to your hypothalamus, the "appetite management center" found in the brain, signaling that your hunger is satisfied. At this point, there will be less chance to overeat. And both psychological and physical appetites will be fulfilled.

❧ HOW MUCH TO EAT

The amount of food you eat should depend, of course, on your body structure and size, your lifestyle and energy demands, and the ideal weight you are trying to achieve or maintain. Through experimentation you will learn how much you can eat and still maintain your proper weight. One thing to remember is that the quantity of food consumed has absolutely no effect per se on the amount of energy which the body will subsequently generate. Rather, it is the quality of food eaten — the right combination of foods eaten during the time of day when the most energy is required to carry out your job effectively. For example, eating a high protein breakfast will give you the energy necessary to perform the morning tasks. Then at noon, a light lunch and later a light dinner should adequately supply the nutritional needs of any person. The late nutritionist, Adelle Davis, suggested in her book, *Let's Eat Right To Keep Fit*: "The general rule is to eat breakfast like a king, lunch like a prince, and dinner like a pauper."[*]

In general, a substantial breakfast is necessary to provide energy through noontime. Many people tend to skip breakfast, take a light lunch, and feast at dinner. This process is healthier in reverse

---

[*] Adelle Davis, *Let's Eat Right To Keep Fit* (New York: Harcourt Brace, 1954), p. 28.

because we normally need energy to perform effectively during the morning hours and a light lunch to continue until dinner. At night, we don't need a lot of energy and thus a heavy dinner contributes to nothing — except possibly insomnia and added weight. Abstaining from breakfast can cause poor concentration, nervousness, and irritability and also tends to result in a low blood sugar level. And low blood sugar levels often encourage the craving for more sugar. If you eat heavily at night, you're likely to experience a feeling of greater energy and will find that a lot of calories are converted into stored-away fat. If you are trying to lose weight, you may still eat three times a day. The key to losing weight is eating only a certain amount of food, which you should determine for yourself.

❧ WHEN TO EAT

One of the best ways to acquire more fat is to come home at 6:00 p.m., head for the kitchen, devour everything edible to satisfy a momentary urge and then wait for dinner later. Unfortunately, many people fall into this trap. Immediately upon walking in the door, you're likely to be tired, if not emotionally drained, from the day's grind and such a time is not the best time to eat dinner. What you can do is engage in other enjoyable activities — anything to divert your attention away from food — and then when dinner comes (best not after 7:00 p.m.) chances are you'll be eating slowly, chewing your food well, and even enjoying the meal. And if you're trying to lose weight, eating slower will have an additional psychological impact. You'll not only be doing yourself a favor, but you will convince everyone else at the table that you're consuming as much as they are. Even if they are eating twice as much, by eating slowly and chewing well you'll keep pace with everyone else and no one will likely comment on your behavior. Whatever your decision, remember that dinner should consist of one "light," but nutritious meal — not snacks after work, dinner an hour later, and snacks before retiring.

❧ *WHAT SHOULD WE EAT*

A healthy skin diet, like any other diet, should be a balanced diet. Often, people get involved in calorie counting and lose focus of their real diet goals altogether. A good diet has more to do with the quality and quantity of food consumed than with the amount of calories consumed per se. A balanced, nutritious diet means eating reasonable, daily portions of the necessary ingredients, including carbohydrates, proteins, and fats. In addition, it is important to have adequate vitamin and mineral elements in the body.

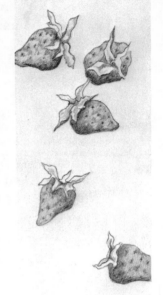

Proteins

Protein cannot be stored in the body and thus needs to be replaced. This nutrient is important to the maintenance and repair of body tissues, as it is vital to the

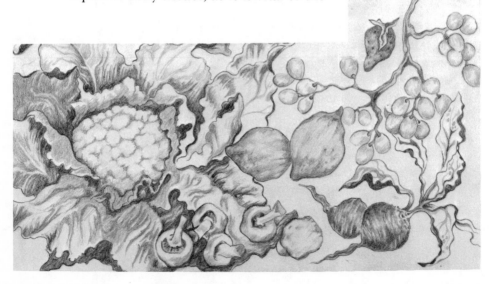

growth of new cells to replace old ones that die. It is also instrumental in the making of hemoglobin (which filters oxygen to cells) and in forming antibodies necessary to resist infection and illness. The best sources of protein include milk, cheese, meat, fish, eggs, nuts, wheat germ, and yogurt.

Carbohydrates

Foodstuffs containing sugar and starches provide carbohydrate. During the digestion process sugars and starches are broken into glucose, an energy source. The central nervous system and your red blood cells need glucose for energy. Some major sources of carbohydrates include brown rice, wheat, rye, barley, whole grain breads and cereals, fresh vegetables and fruit juices, and fresh fruit.

Fats

Fat consumption aids in forming deposits to support vital organs of the body and to provide the body with insulation. Controlling cholesterol consumption is important to good health and replacing saturated fats with unsaturated fats is advised. Essential fatty acids are also necessary for proper functioning of the skin's metabolism. Some of the best sources of unsaturated fatty acids include vegetable oils (safflower oil, corn, sunflower). Also containing fats are eggs, lean meats, nuts, olives, and avocados. Vegetable oils assist in burning up stored fat in the body — ultimately helping in the weight reduction process.

❧ FOODS TO REMEMBER

Cauliflower	Carrots	String Beans
Tomatoes	Corn	Squash
Yams	Asparagus	Broccoli
Garbanzos	Potatoes	Cabbage
Lettuce	Celery	Peas
Bell Peppers	Radishes	Cucumber

All fresh fruits, fruit juices, and vegetable juices.

Meats and Seafood

Fish, chicken, lamb, turkey, lean beef, veal.

Dairy Products

Eggs, cheese, yogurt, cottage cheese

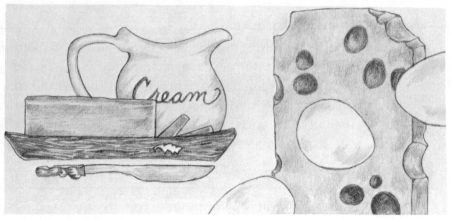

Nuts and Seeds

Raw or dry roasted

Fiber

Oatmeal, wheat bran, rice bran

❧ FOODS TO FORGET

White Sugar Products

Ice Cream	Candy	Soda Pop
Pastries	Cakes	Desserts with meals

Processed Flour Products

Spaghetti	Crackers	Biscuits
Dumplings	Cookies	Cakes
White Breads	Rolls, Buns and	Macaroni
Doughnuts	other bread containing	Pie Crust
	white flour.	

Processed Meat

Weiners	Salami	Corned Beef
Sausages	Bacon	Pastrami
Canned Meat	Lunch Meat	Ground Meat that is not fresh
Pork	Potted Meat	and lean

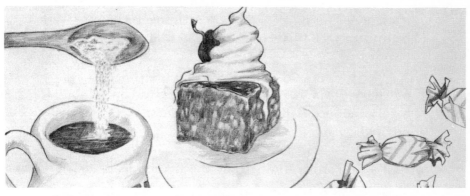

Spiced, Smoked, Pickled and Highly Salted Foods

Tabasco Sauce	Canned Soups	Pickles and pickled foods
Spiced "hot" chili	T.V. Dinners	Smoked meat or fish
Other "hot" sauces	Salted Nuts	

❧ USES OF FRUIT AND VEGETABLE JUICES FOR SKIN

Most raw fruit and vegetable juices contain valuable vitamins, minerals, and enzymes which help promote healthy skin. Juices can be effectively combined with other ingredients and applied to the skin as in the case of homemade masques and facials. Many juices, taken internally, not only enable the development of healthy skin, but also serve as diuretics and thus aid in the elimination of toxic wastes as well. Below is a list of the most popular fruit and vegetable juices which are beneficial for skin health. Along with your personal likes and dislikes, consider the quality and value of various juices before stocking up.

Almond — Almonds contain essential oils and sugars, calcium and vitamins A and B. Almond is beneficial for dry skin and for general body health.

Apple — Apple juice is helpful for skin which is blemished, oily, and irritated. It contains natural sugars, vitamin C, and essential minerals like magnesium, calcium, and iron. It may be used as a light laxative and astringent.

Apricot — This juice is an excellent source of vitamins A and C, and many minerals. It is recommended for all skin types and as a mild laxative.

Banana — Banana is a fruit rich in moisturizing ability. It is good for dry and aged skin and contains vitamins A, C, D, E, magnesium, oils and sugars.

Beet — Beet juice can aid in poor circulation and blood purification.

Cabbage — This juice contains vitamins A, B, C, and D, and minerals such as iron and sulfur. Especially beneficial to oily and blemished skin, it facilitates internal cleansing and healing.

Carrot — Rich in virtually all important vitamins and minerals, this juice acts as moisturizer, promotes cell reproduction, and is excellent for dry, sensitive and mature skin. It contains healthy doses of vitamins A, B, C, D, E, and K, along with many minerals.

Celery — This juice is great for any skin type, contains vitamins A, B, and C and minerals such as calcium, potassium, and phosphorus. It also promotes healthy elimination of bodily waste materials.

Cucumber — Both the skin and juice of cucumber have skin-nourishing ability. Useful for all types of skin, this vegetable contains vitamins A, B, and C and is an effective diuretic.

Dandelion — Dandelion is a valuable blood cleanser and is useful for all skin types. It contains good sources of vitamins A and B, and is high in minerals such as iron, calcium, and potassium.

Grapes — This fruit serves as an aid for blemished skin, is an effective diuretic and contains vitamins A, B, C, and E.

Lemon — Juice of lemon contains a healthy amount of vitamin C and some other vitamins and minerals as well. It has been effectively used as an antiseptic, light bleach, and disinfectant. Most beneficial for oily skin, it may also be applied as a skin toner.

Orange — This juice provides a good dose of vitamins A and C, along with some B. It is often used on oily to normal skin, as an astringent, and an aid for enlarged pores and skin pigmentation problems.

Papaya — This juice has no known skin improvement capability, but has long been used as a digestive aid and has been useful as an internal healing and refreshing agent. Fresh pineapple juice, which also contains a digestive enzyme, is a good digestive aid and body purifier.

Potato — This vegetable is important in the development of healthy skin and is particularly beneficial to aging skin. It has a good supply of vitamin C, potassium, iron, and sugar, and is useful as a diuretic and skin toner.

Spinach — Juice of spinach contains excellent sources of vitamins A, B, and E, along with iron. It is recommended for constipation, dry and blemished skin, and to promote good circulation.

Strawberry — Strawberry is rich in vitamin C and also contains iron and sodium. It is effective not only as a toning agent, but also as an astringent and for normal to oily skin.

Tomato — another good source of vitamin C, tomato also contains vitamins A and B. It is an excellent blood purifier and useful for treatment of oily and blemished skin.

❧ *A WORD ABOUT WATER*

When it comes to health and beauty maintenance, water is an essential, but often neglected part of nutrition. Along with controlling body temperature, water helps dissolve nutrients and facilitates elimination of stored bodily wastes. In cleansing the body of internal pollution, water aids greatly in the development of clear and healthy-looking skin. However, the quality of tap water differs greatly throughout communities and the world. And precisely because tap water consumption often carries with it many health-related risks, it is important to check out the water you are including in your diet.

Studies have shown that water containing only small amounts of the many dangerous chemicals can be cancer-inducing when consumed daily for many years. There are other health hazards associated with polluted water, some of which include behavioral problems (linked to the presence of lead in water) and heart disease and stroke (tied to frequent long-term consumption of "soft water"). Soft water has smaller concentrations of minerals than does hard water, especially magnesium. Magnesium is thought to aid in the reduction of high blood pressure and according to studies, significantly lower levels of magnesium have been found in the hearts of many who died from heart attacks as compared with deaths from other causes. It is believed that the connection between low bodily levels of magnesium interferes in some way with the activity of magnesium-activated heart enzymes and therefore, increases the probability of death when a heart attack is present.

The relationship between water consumption and health maintenance over the long haul is a subject that is just beginning to unfold. Chemicals such as chlorine may destroy germs, but chlorine now has been cited as a possible culprit. Recent investigations show that in reacting with a number of water pollutants, chlorine produces chemical compounds that have been known to increase the chance of bladder cancer and may be linked to other cancers as well.

There are long lists of water pollutants and many others which are likely to be cited in the future. From industrial sites to agricultural areas, the accumulation of toxic wastes continues to threaten the long-term health of those who consume the infested water.

Studies have picked up the traces of agriculturally used chemicals such as fertilizers, pesticides and poisonous sprays, along with many industrial wastes that have been dumped or have otherwise seeped into the water supply. But the list of potential water polluters does not end with agricultural and industrial by-products. Water polluters may include gases and oils from motorboats, metals from water pipes, and innumerable other sources of debris.

The quality of water varies from city to city and region to region and every year or two more studies are confirming a connection between the presence of toxic chemicals and health problems in certain areas. Such water investigations, however, are still very much in the early stages in terms of uncovering a great many of the possible hazards. If you are interested in your health and appearance, it would be wise to look for tap water substitutes.

Appropriate alternatives to tap water include bottled mineral and spring waters. Again, to be sure of what you're getting, read the labels carefully and understand the different grades of bottled water that are available. All commercially marketed bottled waters are not of the same quality. As with tap water, bottled waters vary in their mineral content, alkalinity and acidity, and overall purity.

✠ A FEW SPECIAL FOODS

Wheat Germ

Loaded with many healthy nutrients, wheat germ provides an excellent source of protein, iron and the B and E vitamins. It can be filtered into baked goods and is particularly tasty in breads, biscuits, muffins, and in breakfast foods such as waffles and cereals. A nice topping for salads, soups, eggs and good with fruits, milk, and honey. Wheat germ has been linked to skin breakouts in some people, so keep this in mind as you include it in your diet.

Garlic _____

Garlic, with its diverse uses, acts as a natural body purifier and antiseptic. Rich in sulphur and iodine, garlic improves circulation, guards against varicose veins and aids the digestive system. It also helps control blood pressure. You can choose garlic in natural form (fresh parsley serves to neutralize the odor) or try garlic tablets which are free of odor as well as taste.

Sunflower Seeds _____

Packed with vitamins and minerals and rich in fiber, these gems provide a healthy source of polyunsaturated oil. (High in linoleic acid) An excellent snack food and tasty in salads and cookies. NOTE: Peanuts and other nuts have been cited as containing substances that cause skin breakouts in some cases. Sunflower seeds, as a related food, may have a similar effect in those who are prone to such breakouts.

Honey _____

Pure honey is rich in vitamins B and C and in many minerals (copper, iron, calcium, sodium, potassium). It can replace sugar as a natural sweetening agent and is used also as a laxative.

Yeast _____

Brewers' yeast serves as a valuable natural source of many vitamins (particularly B vitamins) and minerals and is rich in proteins. While the taste may be considered by some as less than palatable, it can easily be added to milk or juices. Yeast flakes and tablets are also available, but brewers' yeast is much richer in nutritional value.

Vegetable Oils _____

The natural vegetable oils are important contributors to health. Rather than fattening, oils such as safflower, corn, soy, and sunflower aid in burning up fat deposits and thus make a positive contribution to the weight reduction process.

❧ *PRACTICAL TIPS FOR MAINTAINING A HEALTHY DIET*

In strengthening oneself for the task of maintaining a balanced diet, consider the following nutritional ideas:

- With the help of your personal physician and/or dietician/ nutritionist, assess your present nutritional needs and design an appropriate dietary plan.
- Do your homework — learn more about the role of diet and nutrition and its potential impact upon your skin as well as your physical/mental health and well-being.
- Consider the opinions of health experts but experiment and ultimately choose your own "best" diet and nutrition strategies.
- Use your imagination and create your own variable menus. Consume small proportions of many different nutritious foods. Once you learn how to maintain your proper weight, an occasional binge won't be detrimental.
- If you're trying to lose weight, think about food only when you are eating — and at that point consider the quality and quantity of what you consume and how it will affect your body.
- Go after what you like but learn not to like those foods which provide little nutritional substance and convert easily into fat.
- Chew your food well and include a variety of wholesome foods as part of your daily diet.
- Don't panic about your weight. If you need to lose some pounds or want to preserve your present condition, follow a consistent and sensible eating routine and don't expect miracles. You didn't balloon overnight and you won't shrink healthfully in a day or two. Remember that frequent and rapid weight gains or losses will hurt, not help, your skin's condition.
- Learn the art of saying "no" to food offers. Regardless of the situation, with a little practice you can learn to stick to your good eating habits while graciously turning away those offers of seconds.

- Avoid becoming obsessed with scale monitoring and calorie-counting. It's really useless. Instead, focus on other more rewarding activities. When you reach your goal, you won't need a scale to confirm it.
- Liquid fasting for twenty-four hours once or twice a month can provide a healthy break for your system. But don't make it a habit. It can be dangerous.
- Include sufficient fiber (roughage) in your diet, keep salt intake to a minimum, and watch your consumption of sugar.
- Try for a healthy balance of carbohydrates, proteins, and fats. Each plays a part in building, repairing, and maintaining a healthy body. Consuming more of one nutrient does not compensate for neglect of the other elements.
- Shop for quality foods, not junk. Learn about what you're consuming by reading food labels. When determining how much protein or carbohydrates to consume, consider the RDA (recommended daily allowance) as devised by the FDA. Keep in mind that there is continual debate on the RDA of vitamins and minerals, so trust your body signals and be your own best guide in selecting foods to meet your lifestyle and energy demands. If you're feeling irritable, exhausted, or nervous you don't need anyone to tell you that you're diet is not up to par.
- Avoid heavy reliance on refined and processed foods, preservatives, and additives. Many foods which contain such chemicals are known to contribute to certain major diseases, particularly if consumed habitually for a long time.
- Consider that little or no breakfast can cause low blood sugar levels, affecting concentration and setting off the junk food binge.
- Stay clear of liquid protein diets and other fads. Such diet schemes are little more than propaganda and may, if used without proper medical supervision, actually endanger your health.

- Remember that how much food you eat as well as when you eat should reflect your personality and lifestyle and energy needs. Develop a sensible attitude toward food, enjoy your meals in a relaxed atmosphere, and learn to create your own original and interesting menus.

✤ EXERCISE AND SKIN HEALTH

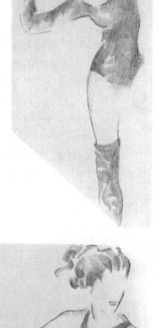

Exercise is not only vital to overall health maintenance, it is also essential to the development of healthy skin. As you exercise, your blood circulation increases and provides fuel and oxygen for the growth of new cells, and for efficient shedding of the dead ones that clog pores and harm the complexion. Vigorous physical conditioning aids in the elimination of waste products built up in different areas of the body, including the skin. And good circulation acquired through regular exercise enables the outer skin to appear fresh and glowing.

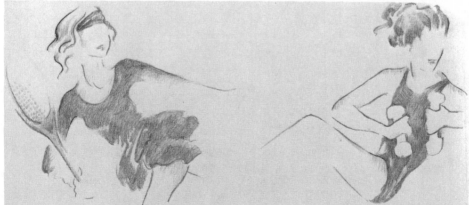

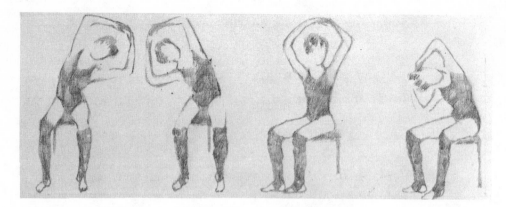

Exercise also influences the skin's condition through the fatty layer and muscles that "fill out" the skin. It helps break down excess fat, improves muscle tone and gives the body a firm appearance. If you lose weight, you must exercise regularly to prevent the skin from sagging. For those who need to gain weight, exercise helps round out and build up the body. Even if you are at a desired weight, exercise enhances the appearance of outer skin by toning and firming it. And as a bonus, when the skin has been sufficiently stimulated and maintained via exercise, you will also find that it is more healthy and youthful-looking.

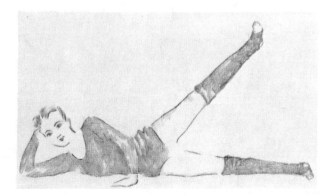

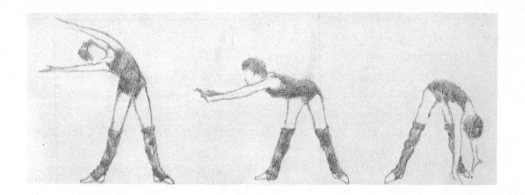

❧ OTHER BENEFITS YOU CAN EXPECT FROM EXERCISE

Decrease Your Appetite and Shed Pounds _____

Exercise is most effective and enjoyable and the least exhaustive when it is done regularly and spontaneously. It improves one's general fitness — toning up muscles, increasing the body's strength and energy and adding renewed vigor and vitality. And it is the only safe and lasting way to lose weight, firm up the body, and maintain the healthy condition.

Studies have shown that regular exercise can actually lower appetite — particularly in people who consistently overeat. Even if the act of exercising doesn't actually reduce your appetite, focusing on some physical activity can be a constructive indulgence and may even serve to keep you out of the kitchen.

Exercise Maintenance Tips

- Stick with it. Decide to begin a program and then do it. Think of how you can best achieve your exercise goals (losing weight, toning and firming muscles, improving stamina and skin tone), what kinds of activity you prefer, and whether you like to work out with friends or alone.
- Choose activities that you enjoy. Don't assume that it's a chore or part-time punishment.
- Develop a schedule for carrying out your exercise. Decide how much exercise, how long, and when in designing your schedule. Keep in mind that to receive real benefits, you should exercise vigorously for at least 30 minutes, three to four times per week.
- Decide which types of exercise are best to accomplish your goals (e.g. swimming, bicycling, jogging, weight lifting, Nautilus machines, ballet, racquet sports, stretching movements).
- Check with your physician before embarking on a strenuous exercise regimen. You will be advised to follow exercise guidelines appropriate for your physical health and condition. If you have any handicap or disorder such as diabetes, high blood pressure, asthma, heart disease, or other problems, it is especially important to seek medical advice regarding exercises.
- Start slowly and build up your exercise time as you increase your strength and endurance. Don't quit too soon, but don't overdo it, either.
- Be patient and consistent. The best results take time — and effort.
- After you've designed and begun to implement your exercise plan, remember that the key to attaining and maintaining the rewards of exercise are motivation and willpower, patience and persistence, and optimistic realism.

6. The Role of Vitamins

Vitamins are important in the control and regulation of body processes. They contribute to cellular development, help to ensure a healthy nervous system, aid in the digestive process and they help us convert food into actual energy. Most vitamins come from food, but others are actually manufactured in the body. If you are eating a well-balanced diet, chances are you're obtaining most all of the necessary vitamins needed to ensure maximum wellness. However, you may need a vitamin supplement or supplements upon occasion. Know what you need and avoid taking large doses of synthetic vitamins unless you are under medical supervision. There's still a lot to be learned regarding the use of vitamin supplements and their subsequent impact on the body. Various kinds of side effects such as skin eruptions or kidney problems can result from misuse or overdose of vitamin supplements. Try to satisfy your vitamin and mineral requirements by relying on natural food sources and by sticking to a nutritious diet. Following is a list of the most important vitamins and minerals.

Vitamin A

Vitamin A is important for strong bones and teeth, good vision, and in maintaining firm, smooth skin. It helps in the building of body cells and in keeping hair and nails healthy.
Sources: green and yellow vegetables, eggs, liver, dairy products, carrots, tomatoes.

[83]

Vitamin B Complex

The vitamin B family is composed of a number of different vitamins all of which work together intricately. The vitamin B complex aids the nervous system process and is involved in the production of hemoglobin (red blood cells). It also serves to ensure that hair, skin and eyes are healthy. Practically all of the vitamins in this family can be found in wheat germ and brewer's yeast.

Vitamins included in the B complex are: thiamine (B_1), riboflavin (B_2), pyridoxine (B_6), cyanocobalamin (B_{12}), folic acid, pantothenic acid, niacin, choline, inositol, and biotin.

Thiamine (B_1) — Necessary for proper digestion, elimination and helps nerves remain healthy.
Sources: whole grains, wheat germ, molasses, brewer's yeast, eggs.

Riboflavin (B_2) — This element is a valuable aid in keeping skin, eyes, and nerves in healthy condition. And it aids in the metabolism of fat, carbohydrates, and proteins.
Sources: avocados, pork, turkey, yogurt, leafy green vegetables, wheat germ, brewer's yeast, milk, eggs, and liver are all excellent sources of riboflavin.

Pyridoxine (B_6) — Participates in the metabolism (utilization) of fats and proteins, and is important for good functioning of the nerves and muscles.
Sources: wheat germ, whole grains, brewer's yeast, green vegetables, nuts, milk.

Cyanocobalamin (B_{12}) — Instrumental in the development of red blood cells.
Sources: milk, fish, eggs, liver.

Folic Acid — Important for the development of red blood cells.
Sources: milk, fish eggs, liver.

Pantothenic Acid — Important for proper functioning of the digestive system and a participant in carbohydrate metabolism.
Sources: brewer's yeast, leafy green vegetables, organ meats.

Vitamin C

Vitamin C helps the body utilize other vitamins and minerals and aids in the assimilation of medications. It is vital in maintaining the good health of skin, bones, teeth, tendons, blood vessels walls, collagen, and cartilage. And it is well-known that Vitamin C does play a significant role in preventing colds and lessening the symptoms of a cold once it has set in. For the appearance of skin, Vitamin C is invaluable because it is important in the production of collagen, the essential protein that keeps the body together. A deficiency of Vitamin C will affect the collagen function and the result will be skin that is lifeless — blotchy, sagging, wrinkled, and perhaps even filled with broken capillaries. Vitamin C is so essential for healthy skin that without it, the chances of developing acne, flaky and dry skin, dermatitis and related problems increase greatly.

Your intake of Vitamin C depends on your metabolism and lifestyle, among other things. Each of us needs Vitamin C to protect our skin and to prevent premature aging. And if you do find Vitamin C helpful in preventing and fighting the common cold, don't take aspirin as it completely neutralizes the effect of Vitamin C.

A good source of Vitamin C can be found in rose hips, citrus fruits, tomatoes, leafy green vegetables, and many other vegetables.

Vitamin D

Vitamin D is important for strong teeth and bones and is manufactured by the body, when it is exposed to sunlight. Necessary for the body's proper utilization of calcium and phosphorous.
Sources: milk, eggs, and fish liver oil.

Vitamin E

Essential for healthy functioning of the endocrine glands, this vitamin is needed by the blood vessels and is able to store oxygen. Although, scientific support is still lacking, many people have found Vitamin E to be an aid in healing certain skin disorders. Others have found that Vitamin E aggravates acne and when applied topically to the skin, the vitamin has been known to cause allergic reactions.

Sources: sunflower seeds, vegetable oils, wheat germ, spinach, celery.

Niacin

Aids in breakdown of sugar and starches to release energy. Helps nervous system and contributes to skin, mouth, and digestive functions.

Sources: mushrooms, liver, brewer's yeast, broccoli, peas, heart, kidneys, egg yolks.

Choline

Necessary for utilization of cholesterol and in fat distribution throughout the body.

Sources: wheat germ, nuts, liver, leafy green vegetables.

Inositol

Works intricately with choline, particularly in the fat distribution process and in protecting the liver. Also aids in the absorption of Vitamin E.

Sources: brewer's yeast, wheat germ, whole grains, liver, fruit.

Biotin

Important for the digestion and assimilation of fats and apparently a contributor to good mental health.

Sources: wheat germ, liver, brewer's yeast.

Vitamin F

This vitamin in combination with cholesterol and proteins is so essential in the formation of bodily structures that without them there would be no life. Among other functions, this vitamin aids in the development of healthy membranes (in which individual cells are enclosed). When the membrane is defective, weak, or non-existent, the cell dies. Vitamin F also produces myelin, a protein

substance that protects the major nerves. This vitamin is also known as unsaturated fatty acids and is essential for the distribution of calcium and the absorption of fat soluble vitamins A, D, E, and K.
Sources: pure vegetable oils, milk, butter, and wheat germ.

Vitamin K

Vitamin K is manufactured by the body, needed for proper blood coagulation and important in the prevention of hemorrages.
Sources: cauliflower, cabbage, green peas, broccoli, lettuce, spinach, all green leafy vegetables, eggs, soybean oil, and blackstrap molasses.

Vitamin P

Commonly known as the bioflavonoids, Vitamin P works along with Vitamin C in the maintenance of healthy capillaries.
Sources: leafy green vegetables, prunes and citrus fruits, rose hips, and tomatoes.

Minerals

Minerals are vital in maintaining a healthy nervous system and work together with vitamins in the various metabolic functions. They are also important in maintaining and regulating water balance in the body.

Calcium

Necessary for the building of strong bones and teeth, and a valuable aid in promoting good sleep and relaxation. Serves to alleviate muscle cramps and tension.
Sources: milk, watercress, carrots, yogurt, molasses, Swiss, parmesan, and yellow cheeses.

Phosphorus

Works together with calcium and is an important contributor in converting protein to amino acids.
Sources: fish, meat, whole grains, poultry.

Iodine

Serves as a catalyst and is necessary for proper regulation of the thyroid gland — the gland which is connected to the maintenance of body weight.
Sources: shellfish, fish, spinach, cranberries.

Iron

Important in the building of red blood corpuscles and is essential in carrying oxygen to different parts of the body. Although iron is important for all, women often need an extra dose.
Sources: whole grains, liver, eggs, wheat germ, oysters, dried fruits, molasses, dried yeast.

Sodium (salt)

Necessary for the control of body fluids and aids in the elimination of carbon dioxide.
Sources: oysters, clams, white fish, spinach, watercress, wheat germ, molasses, celery.

Magnesium

Helps in the prevention of cramps and in the protection of nerves. Serves also as a synthesizer of proteins in the body.
Sources: clams, nuts, natural honey, whole grains, green leafy vegetables.

Potassium

Helps in regulating the body's water balance and has a direct impact on the nervous system.
Sources: molasses, citrus fruits, paprika, whole grains, bananas, fish, meat.

A number of other minerals are also needed by the body. Some of these include copper, sulphur, zinc, fluoride, and manganese.

7. Facing Up to common Skin Disorders

When you adhere to the five skin care steps outlined in Chapters 2 and 3 — cleansing, exfoliation, toning, moisturizing, and stimulating — you are completing an important part of the total skin care regimen. Some skin disorders still may persist despite the practice of a regular skin care routine. As mentioned previously, other factors such as proper nutrition, exercise, environmental elements, and personal habits also influence the skin's condition. However, some of the most common skin problems can often be controlled, if not eliminated, by understanding the underlying causes and taking regular preventive measures.

ACNE

Causes

Acne is most common among adolescents, but many adults are also faced with this skin disorder. Although the underlying cause of acne is not completely understood, most experts agree that the condition is accompanied by overactive oil glands, which are also affected by certain hormonal changes in the body, stress, diet, climatic and genetic factors. During the teenage years levels of testosterone and progesterone — two hormones vital to the growth process —increase greatly and at the same time, these hormones tend to stimulate the oil glands toward overproduction of oil. The oil and dead skin cells build up in the follicle (the pore) and eventually the result is whiteheads and blackheads, pimples, or even cysts.

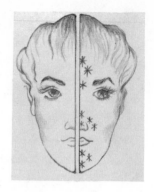

When dead cells collect over the follicle opening and oil accumulates inside, a visible lump may appear on the skin's surface. Since the build-up of dead skin blocks the release of the lump, it remains trapped internally and forms a whitehead. Blackheads, as they appear on the skin's surface, are actually a mass of dead skin cells which have combined with oil and other natural material. As this mass moves to the surface, a buildup of melanin pigment contributes to its dark color. Pimples originate as the follicle walls are weakened by excessive oil, cell build-up and bacteria. As the follicle starts to break open, oil, dead cells, and debris flow into the skin's dermal layer and the result is an inflammation on the outer skin. If the follicle spills an excess of matter that penetrates deep into the dermis, a wall may form around this leakage and result in a more advanced eruption known as a cyst. On the skin's surface, a cyst will appear as a large lump under the skin and will often require medical treatment.

Negative or prolonged stress may aggravate an existing case of acne, but stress alone has rarely been cited as a primary cause of this condition. The link between diet and acne is still being explored, but some foods are thought to be more connected with acne than others. For example, the general feeling is that if you have acne or may be susceptible to it, you should either eliminate or greatly reduce your intake of items containing high levels of iodine, androgen, and bromide (refer to Chapter 5). For acne management, Vitamins A, B, and C and an adequate supply of zinc are especially important nutritional requirements.

Along with the above factors, acne may also be affected by climatic and genetic conditions. Extremely hot and humid weather can accelerate oil gland production. And although exposure to sun may bring about an improvement in acne in some people, others report that their acne condition increases after being out in the sun. Acne is not a condition that is inherited per se, but if your parents — either one or both — were plagued with acne, there is a good possibility that you may also encounter the problem.

Treatment and Prevention _____

A common and often effective approach to acne includes the application of Vitamin A acid directly to the skin. It is also known as retinoic acid and sold under the name of Retin-A. This prescription only medication comes in lotion, gel, or cream form and works by preventing the excess growth of cells around the follicle and by peeling away layers of old cells that tend to clog the pores. With the initial treatment, Vitamin A acid can make the acne worse, but after several weeks it curbs the oiliness and breakouts, and the skin appears smoother and less troubled. When Vitamin A acid is applied properly and consistently, the results can be excellent.

Like Vitamin A acid, benzoyl peroxide has been very successful in controlling and clearing acne. In addition to peeling the surface and loosening impactations, this topical agent also fights bacteria deep into the pore. It is used to treat all stages of acne and is available in many over-the-counter formulas and by prescription. Different products vary in their degree of effectiveness.

One of the most recent discoveries for severe acne is the acne pill called Accutane. It is used to treat advanced cases of acne, but is not usually recommended for mild to moderate cases. Like other drugs, Accutane has its drawbacks. Significant side effects include drying of the body's mucous membranes, nosebleeding, drying of the lips and even the possibility of birth defects if used during or near pregnancy. Accutane is also expensive and its side effects are still being explored.

Topical antibiotics are also useful as antibacterial agents in controlling acne. Both erythromycin lotion and clindomycin (Cleocin-T™) lotion can be very effective and are often prescribed in conjunction with Vitamin A acid or benzoyl peroxide. Oral clindomycin has been associated with diarrhea and colitis, but such side effects are rare when it is used topically. Certain erythromycin lotions may contain laureth-4, a substance that is comedogenic.

In some cases dermatologists still prescribe tetracycline (an antibiotic) to combat the acne. This drug has been successful in reducing acne by changing the chemical structure of fatty acids in the skin so that the oil glands produce less oil and there is less cell build-up around the follicle.

Another technique is the use of cortisone, usually injected directly into a cyst. This drug acts to suppress the inflammation within the cyst without resulting in scar tissue. Although effective in controlling many skin problems, cortisone can have side effects with prolonged use and should always be used only with the advice and monitoring of a physician.

For large cysts, a slush bath consisting of powdered carbon dioxide, acetone, and powdered sulfur is sometimes applied to the entire face and left on for about 15-20 minutes. After rinsing, an acne lotion is applied. This treatment facilitates peeling of the skin's outer surface and helps to reduce acne scars and formation of new growths. The technique should be administered by a dermatologist as incorrect use can result in severe damage to the skin.

Occasionally a dermatologist will recommend that a cyst be lanced or cut open in order to encourage healing. The process involves a tiny incision into the top of the cyst. The cut creates a small hole and the cyst can release its contents and enable the skin to start healing.

Zinc tablets are also useful in controlling acne in some people. When taken regularly in a dosage appropriate for one's skin and body, (75-125 mg. per day is common) zinc may help reduce the occurrence of skin eruptions. If zinc tablets have been taken for two to three months with no results, then you should assume they will not help.

X-ray therapy and ultraviolet treatment are now considered obsolete in the fight against acne. X-ray therapy, was often used for advanced acne to reduce the activity of the oil glands by destroying its active cells. The idea was that less oil would be released by the sebaceous glands. It is now recognized, however, that the X-rays are harmful to the skin and have been tied to the occurrence of skin cancer in later life.

Ultraviolet treatment has also been used to control acne. It helps bring about peeling of the outer layer of skin, but must be used about three to four times a week for several weeks to be effective. This technique is now considered outmoded as the cost can be fairly high, and certain risks (such as burns) are associated with home treatment. Many other methods available today (as mentioned in this section) are more effective, and less costly and hazardous.

To control acne it is imperative to keep the skin clean. This cleansing routine should be carried out with the advice of a trusted dermatologist who will suggest cleansers that are appropriate for your skin's condition. Regardless of the cleansing agent selected, it is important to have very clean hands and also to steam your face one to two times per week to release internal waste matter.

Some treatments are available for diminishing the effect of scars left by acne breakouts. Such techniques include dermabrasion (discussed under Dermatological Treatments in Chapter 8), chemical peeling, and cosmetic surgery. These techniques, if necessary, must be performed by a highly competent and experienced dermatologist or plastic surgeon.

✣ LINES AND WRINKLES

Causes

Most women over twenty-five have at least some fine lines on their face. Usually these lines first appear around the eyes, forehead, and in the nose/mouth area. Such lines are not necessarily indications of aging but often are related to general wear and tear on the skin and overexposure to sun. Both of these factors can cause the collagen fibers to become frayed, disordered, and to change shape. Wrinkle-free skin is a result of collagen that has retained its order and flexibility. Collagen is a protein substance that makes up a large part of the dermis and is responsible for the appearance of youthful-looking skin. After many years of constant motion and facial expression the collagen fibers gradually begin to lose some of their earlier resilience and fine lines emerge.

Excessive exposure to sun will only accelerate the appearance of fine lines and wrinkles and the damage is irreversible. Some women also have a genetic susceptibility to premature wrinkling of the skin. In addition, rapid and frequent weight gain and loss, prolonged stress, over-massaging and creaming of the face, and long-term skin folding as a result of sleeping on one side of the face may also encourage wrinkle development.

Treatment and Prevention

Once pronounced wrinkles have set in, there is little outside of cosmetic surgery that can be done to improve the skin's appearance. There are many techniques promoted to diminish or remove wrinkles, from facial peels and silicone therapy to various cream formulas. At the present time, however, the only procedure that is known to significantly improve the wrinkled skin's appearance is cosmetic surgery. A face lift operation is the procedure used to lift and smooth skin over the entire face. Some plastic surgeons may recommend surgery on specific areas of the face as compared to a complete face lift. However, the cost of several spot operations performed separately usually exceeds the price of a complete face lift. A chemical peel may be suggested in place of or in combination with a face lift. (See Chapter 8).

Prevention of premature wrinkling is a long-term process that should begin in early life. If you avoid overexposure to sun, stay away from smoking and heavy drinking, minimize exaggerated facial expressions and massage, and have maintained good nutrition and skin cleansing habits, you will be rewarded with nice skin for many years longer than if you have previously abused your skin. Finally, regardless of how well you care for your face, the day will come when wrinkles appear. At this point, you may want to consider a form of cosmetic surgery such as a face lift or chemical peel.

❧ *FRECKLES, KERATOSES, AND RED LINES*

Causes

Freckles are groups of cells that have acquired too much melanin, the dark brown pigment of the skin. As a result of excessive sun, freckles usually become visible in childhood.

Solar keratoses appear as scaly, brownish-red lesions in areas that have been overexposed to the sun. They often occur in clusters and are more prevalent on fair-skinned people. These spots, like liver spots and freckles, can mar the skin and give it an aged look beyond its years.

Red lines (telangiectasia) in the nose or cheek areas appear as a result of broken blood vessels. The exact cause of such red lines is not exactly clear, but there are a number of underlying factors that seem to promote the development of this condition. Genetic susceptibility toward broken red lines in the skin, a traumatic blow to the skin that results in the breakage of small blood vessels, or high blood pressure (extreme enough to burst small blood vessels) may all facilitate the appearance of little red lines. Other factors such as heavy drinking (large quantities of alcohol can expand the blood vessels to the point of bursting), and frequent exposure to warmth, including open fires, electric heaters, and sunlight can cause the small, delicate blood vessels to rupture and show up as red lines. There is also evidence that constant overindulgence in heavily spiced foods may encourage this skin problem. Finally, the burden of pregnancy can cause poor circulation and excessive pressure on blood vessels in the legs. This strain can ultimately result in varicose veins as well as red lines on the legs.

Treatment and Prevention

For the treatment of freckles, techniques such as dermabrasion, a mild superficial chemical peel or chemical freeze can be effective. Once the freckles are diminished or removed, they will again return if the skin is exposed to sun. A good sunscreen should always be used even when sun exposure time is limited. Dermatologists may sometimes prescribe a bleach cream in combination with another technique to lighten the freckles. However, freckle bleaching creams and lotions purchased over-the-counter usually have very little, if any, effect, on the appearance and removal of freckles. A hydroquinone preparation applied regularly for several months after the freckles have been treated with one of the techniques noted above, may be helpful in lightening the spots or even clearing them substantially. However, if such a preparation is used, it's important to keep the treated area away from sun exposure, to be aware of possible skin irritation that might occur, and to remember that the safety of applying this preparation during pregnancy has not been determined.

Solar keratoses can be successfully treated by freezing with carbon dioxide or liquid nitrogen (also referred to as cryotherapy), by electrodesiccation and curettage, by treatment with trichloroacetic acid (TCA) and phenol, or with 5-Fluorouracil.

Cryotherapy is often the treatment of choice as it is relatively inexpensive (usually covered under insurance) and it is simple, quick and effective. This resurfacing method is usually suggested for a small number of lesions; scarring is rare.

When stubborn keratoses cannot be eliminated with cryotherapy, electrodesiccation with curettage may be used. An electric needle is used to desiccate the lesion area and the lesion is scraped off with a curette. The scraped particle then serves as a biopsy specimen for skin cancer testing. The healing process is longer than with cryotherapy and a scar usually results. The type of scar varies from lesion to lesion and person to person. For multiple keratoses, dermatologists may suggest chemical treatment with 5-Fluorouracil. This chemical is thought to destroy damaged cells without causing any harm at all to normal cells and it should be used only under the supervision of a physician. Finally, TCA and phenol have been used to treat some keratoses, but these methods are seldom recommended because of the discomfort and complications involved.

Little red lines can be treated by cauterization. This process involves applying an electric needle or electrosurgical tip to the end of the tiny red line. The electric current seals off the blood vessel and the visible red lines disappear from view. Some vessels may reopen and appear again and a second treatment can then be performed. After this treatment, red lines may continue to appear in other places unless the original cause of such lines has also been confronted. Therefore, in order to prevent against the onset of red lines, it is necessary to be aware of the underlying factors that promote this condition (e.g. high blood pressure, excessive exposure to sun and warmth, heavy drinking), and to eliminate the causes of this condition before undergoing treatment.

❧ BROWN SPOTS

Causes

Brown spots or liver spots (technically known as lentigines) represent changes in the pigmentation of the skin. They appear in all sizes and are most often found in areas frequently exposed to sun such as hands and the face. Thin-skinned and blond people are especially prone to developing these dark spots which occur as a result of both age and sun exposure.

Treatment and Prevention

Dermatologists can remove liver spots by applying liquid nitrogen, frozen carbon dioxide, or the electric needle. Skin peeling and/or bleach cream may also be recommended for elimination of these spots. Although brown spots can usually be removed successfully, there is little that can be done internally to prevent them. However, if you are prone to this skin disorder, you must stay out of the sun in order to protect against new spots developing. Once removed, the spots usually do not return as long as your skin is protected from the sun.

✺ *CELLULITE*

Causes

A universally accepted definition of cellulite is yet to evolve. According to one line of thought (many noted physicians subscribe to this belief) cellulite is just pure and ordinary fat that can be prevented or eliminated largely through a controlled diet and vigorous exercise. Other physicians consider cellulite to be a gelatin-type substance made up of fat, water, and waste materials that accumulates and lodges in areas such as the thighs, knees, hips, and upper arms and back. From this point of view, cellulite is caused, in part, by poor circulation and improper elimination. There are still other ideas about cellulite among professionals in the health field. Some believe it was "invented" in order to defraud the public. In general, there are two types of so-called cellulite. Soft cellulite resembles cottage cheese in appearance when pressed and the hard type looks similar to orange peel when squeezed.

Treatment and Prevention

Although there are many advertised anti-cellulite techniques that claim to cure this problem, they should be viewed with caution. If there were a sure-fire cure for this problem called cellulite then it would be widely available, well-proven, and well-known. As it stands, the problem can be largely treated and reduced through self-care at home. However, there is no easy or completely effective method available to remove these fatty pockets. Since individuals respond differently to different techniques, it's important to experiment and ultimately uncover what works best for you. The guidelines listed below will help break down those difficult fatty deposits. And if you're not yet bothered by "cellulite," practicing these suggestions will aid in preventing the development of this condition.

Diet

Being diet-wise is one indisputable precaution in the fight against cellulite. A typical anti-cellulite diet would be made up of four to six mini meals per day including foods such as fresh, raw fruits and vegetables, poultry, lean meat, eggs, plain yogurt, skim milk, salads with pure vegetable oil dressings, low-fat cheese, juices, brewer's yeast, wheat germ, and six to eight glasses of water per day (between meals).

The fish, poultry and lean meat should be prepared by roasting or baking and consumed in moderation.

Unprocessed and unsalted nuts and seeds may be taken with meals or snacks.

Exercise

Along with good nutrition comes regular and vigorous exercise. Spot exercising which focuses on particular cellulite areas is important along with swimming, biking, jogging (for thighs), aerobics, and yoga. Working out on Nautilus or other equipment can help firm, tone, and ultimately break down some of the cellulite.

Massage

Massage can be beneficial as it aids in breaking down the fatty deposits which appear as cellulite. Stimulating dry skin is also helpful in forcing blood and nutrients to the skin's surface. Such skin stimulation can be accomplished by using a body brush, loofah, or similar device. Try massaging the affected areas with mustard oil. Rub in well all over the affected area, then work on particular problem spots. Leave on at least an hour and then take a warm bath spiced with epsom salt. During the bath use your loofah to massage the cellulite spots.

Saunas

Saunas also aid in cleansing the body of toxins and waste materials through perspiration. Such excretion further assists in the "cellulite" elimination process. The careful use of saunas, however, should be restricted to those without high blood pressure, heart disease or other major health problems.

Calming and Cleansing

Proper breathing, relaxation, and rest are very necessary in avoiding destructive stress effects and in maintaining good body circulation. Along this line, it is helpful to enjoy frequent baths spiced with oils and herbs and to partake of herbal teas. Although this routine may provide only psychological benefits, it will aid in reducing stress and tension, which can affect the development of cellulite. There are herbal teas which tend to act as a diuretic and thus encourage further excretion of waste materials and excess water. Such teas are tasty and free of many chemicals found in over-the-counter diuretics and laxatives. However, herbal tea and supplement products should be used in moderation as their safety has not been fully established.

Diuretic Tests

Herbs such as asparagus, corn silk, and chamomile can be used sparingly in teas to help facilitate proper elimination and breakdown of cellulite.

Diuretic Tea of Cornsilk

Add 2 ounces of corn silk to 1 quart of very hot water. Bring to a boil. Spice with honey and lemon, if desired.

Diuretic Tea of Dandelion

Mix 1 ounce of dandelion with 1 ounce chamomile and 1 ounce comfrey leaf. As needed add 2 tablespoons of herb mixture to 1½ cups boiling water. Strain and add a touch of lemon.

8. Dermatological Treatments for certain Skin Problems

Skin care is a very personal endeavor and different people prefer different types of treatment. Furthermore, what works for you may not be effective for your mom, girlfriend, or daughter. Some people prefer traditional procedures such as dermatological consultation which may result in a skin improvement plan that includes frequent intake of prescribed drugs, application of drying lotions, ointments or other such products, chemical or surgical manipulation of the skin, or even a combination of all these alternatives. Depending on the type of skin problem, some dermatologists will help design a simple home skin-care program that you can follow with a minimum of prescribed products.

Other current skin-care methods that are frequently utilized include those which focus on nutrition, lifestyle/stress and self-care, and home-administered skin-improvement techniques.

Each of the above methods has its place in skin-care, but extreme reliance on any one method for a long period of time is likely to do your skin more harm than good. As in other endeavors, moderation is the key. If, for example, you believe that stress is the sole cause of your frequent skin breakouts and thus pay no attention to your nutritional intake, the types of products you apply to your skin, or the effects on your skin of prescribed drugs, you are seeing only part of the problem and will certainly not be able to find the right answer. Since your "right" answer may be different from your neighbors, it's best to look at all the possible causes as well as the existing range of methods to deal with them.

[101]

The type of treatment as well as the time at which you should seek treatment depend on the nature of the problem. Not all skin disorders need chemical or surgical attention. The dermatological techniques described in this section and the skin disorders discussed in Chapter 7 provide examples of skin problems that may be treated via dermatological procedures.

This section is not meant to be a treatise on current dermatological procedures but rather a brief description of some of the most common treatments used in skin care today.

✣ FACIALS

Facials can be done at home, by well-trained cosmeticians, or by dermatologists. There are many different types of facials, many of which can benefit the skin. Refer to Chapter 10 for facials that can be prepared at home.

✣ CRYOTHERAPY

Freezing with liquid nitrogen (LN_2) or carbon dioxide (CO_2), is also called cryotherapy. These techniques are used to treat solar keratoses (sun-induced skin lesions that sometimes develop into cancer), freckles, liver spots, and related skin problems. Liquid nitrogen is now more widely used, as it is easier to administer than is carbon dioxide. On the whole, cryotherapy is effective, quick, and often covered under insurance. It is almost painless and very rarely results in any scarring. In rare cases a tiny white spot may remain at the treatment site. Cryotherapy is applied in the dermatologist's office and does not require medication or any confinement.

✣ FACE PEELS

Chemical face peels have been used since the 1950's and are primarily designed to improve the appearance of sun-damaged or aged skin. The procedure has been generally successful in treating large quantities of solar keratoses, freckles, and irregular increases in pigmentation. The chemical peel can be time-consuming, expensive, and more uncomfortable than cryotherapy. In fact, the peel is considered similar to a second-degree burn and thus is temporarily painful. If administered correctly, the phenol facial peel can be effective in diminishing wrinkles and other skin problems related to sun and aging. However, there are known risks and possible complications. Such side effects include uneven pigmentation, scarring, occurrence of milia (tiny white "cysts"), cold sores, or fever blisters. With phenol face peels, there is also a more serious side effect. Although uncommon, if administered carelessly, there is the rare, but real possibility of systemic poisoning. Phenol poisoning may lead to a depressed central nervous system and may contribute to a temperature decrease, cardiac irregularity, and respiratory arrest. Phenol can poison the heart and severely affect the kidneys. The possibility of death from a chemical peel is certainly not common but can occur if too large an area is treated in a rapid and less than cautious manner.

❧ TRICHLORACETIC ACID PEELS (TCA)

This chemical is used in varying concentrations to treat problems such as chloasma (mask of pregnancy) and melasma, a side effect of oral contraceptives. For these problems, a concentration of 15-20% is generally applied. Sun-damaged skin may also be helped by a 25-35% concentration. Since this is a more concentrated peel it is also a deeper peel, more uncomfortable, and thus takes longer to heal. A 50% solution is occasionally used for treatment of some wrinkles and freckles. While this TCA peel does not penetrate as deep as the phenol peel, it has been shown to provide good results and with less potential for side effects. TCA is not poisonous to organs such as the heart and kidneys, and death is not known to be a possibility. Swelling, infection, and pigmentation problems are the most serious complications that have been reported. And as would be expected, the stronger the solution, the greater the chance of complication. However, reactions vary from person to person. Overall, facial peels seem to be most effective in correcting spotty and irregular pigmentation and in the treatment of fine wrinkles.

✤ *FACELIFTS*

This method of skin manipulation is usually applied to alter sagging and wrinkled-looking skin, particularly the deeper wrinkles. However, this procedure is not usually as effective in diminishing wrinkles on the forehead, eyelids and upper lip area. A chemical peel is of more value in correcting these areas.

✤ *ELECTRODESICCATION AND CURETTAGE*

Keratoses sometimes are extremely thick and cannot be treated successfully with cryotherapy. When this is the case, electrodesiccation with curretage is recommended. An electric needle is used to desiccate (dry out) a particular area. The lesion is then scraped off with a currete and the scraped specimen can be used in a biopsy test for skin cancer. Although this process is basically painless, it takes longer to heal than cryotherapy and usually leaves a scar. Electrodessication is also used to treat broken capillaries.

✤ *5-FLUOROUCIL*

Another chemical treatment used to reduce or eliminate keratoses is *5-Fluorouracil* (5-F.U.). In contrast to trichloracetic acid or phenol, 5-F.U. is known for its effectiveness in destroying damaged cells without harming normal cells. It has the advantage of killing damaged cells that have not yet developed into visible skin lesions, but would eventually surface and require treatment. 5-F.U. is applied at home (under the supervision of a physician) and is usually recommended for people with multiple keratoses. Although there are no major side effects reported from this treatment, the skin is red and crusty during the process of treatment, and the formation of scabs is common. Once the treatment is completed, the skin becomes smoother than before, with keratoses eliminated. The skin returns to its normal color and texture and usually appears younger, with fine wrinkles and other indications of aging reduced. The period of healing is about 7-8 weeks from initial treatment. 5-F.U. is popular, both because of its success rate and the fact that it is an inexpensive route.

DERMABRASION

This method is being used for treatment of scars left by acne and also for problems related to aging and sun-damaged skin. It can be used over most parts of the body and is considered a much more complicated and expensive treatment than 5-F.U. Dermabrasion is not normally recommended except in cases of severely sun-damaged skin, where keratoses have returned after being treated with 5-F.U. Such cases are rare, however, and today dermabrasion is advised primarily for treating acne scars. When it is used occasionally for the treatment of keratoses, there is less chance of keratoses returning than with 5-F.U., if the patient is careful in using sunscreens and avoiding sun exposure. Dermabrasion is helpful in diminishing the appearance of wrinkles and aged skin and appears to penetrate deeper into the tissue. When administered correctly, dermabrasion can result in skin that is much smoother, softer and younger looking than before. Unfortunately, side effects are common and more complicated with dermabrasion than with 5-F.U. If the treatment has penetrated the tissue too deeply, the result can be scarring. An increase or decrease in pigmentation (hyperpigmentation) is another possible result, as is infection, bleeding, and occurrence of milia. Although the time required for healing varies from person to person, the process can be long in comparison to other methods, and especially so if side effects should occur. Also dermabrasion is usually not covered by insurance, unless performed for medical reasons. Finally, the end result is uncertain and varies from person to person, depending on many factors such as skin type, severity of skin problems, expertise and skill of the performing physician, and the patient's understanding and willingness to cooperate throughout the healing process and afterwards.

SILICONE

Silicone is yet another method desired by some for the treatment of wrinkles, scars, or for corrective treatment on those who have suffered facial disfigurations as a result of disease or accident. Still a controversial method of treatment, silicone is not approved by the

FDA, but is often used as an experimental investigational treatment. However, there are physicians who do silicone injections on patients desiring this method. Although this drug has been around for a long time, there is still much to learn about its application and effectiveness and its possible side effects. For the treatment of skin problems, there are other methods which can be used safely and effectively and which are FDA approved. Such methods include those previously described.

❧ *ZYDERM™ COLLAGEN IMPLANT*

Another method currently popular and used to remove wrinkles, scars, and other skin disfigurations is the *zyderm™ collagen implant*. Although many cosmetics now include collagen as an ingredient, it is not effective when applied to the skin, since it cannot be absorbed into the skin structure. Injectible collagen is produced from cow collagen and must be processed to insure its safe and effective use. Collagen is most frequently sought for its effectiveness in diminishing wrinkles and other apparent signs of aging. However, it is not considered a substitute for facelifts, peels, or dermabrasion. It is often used along with these other techniques to provide additional facial improvement.

Current information on collagen suggests that it is safe, with few side effects. However, collagen implants is fairly new and only limited data regarding its long-term effects is available. It is not advised for pregnant women, as possible effects have not yet been established. Like any other new medical technique or drug, its use should be considered carefully. If you are thinking about a collagen implant, first consult your skin specialist, a dermatologist, plastic surgeon, or ear-throat-and-nose specialist. A medical history check should be done to see if you would be a suitable candidate for this type of procedure. The presence of certain diseases in you or your family may mean that the procedure would be risky and unsuitable for you. Your physician will also perform a skin test to see if you are sensitive to collagen. Although the percentage of skin test failures is low, it's necessary to find out if an allergic reaction develops.

Whether or not collagen is your treatment of choice should also depend on the nature of your skin problem. To date, collagen has been most effective in diminishing wrinkles and scars from acne, accidents, or surgery. Should you pass the preliminaries and you are advised that a collagen implant would be both safe and suitable, you must then shop carefully to find a physician who is sympathetic to your best interests and who is highly skilled in this procedure.

ELECTROSURGICAL TIP

The electrosurgical tip or electric needle is used in the treatment of telangiectasia, a cluster of small blood vessels that have become dilated and appear as "spiders." This problem occurs frequently on the cheeks (in other areas as well) and can be treated successfully, with immediate results. In some cases, more than one treatment is required to eliminate the "spidered" appearance.

SALT WATER INJECTION

Blood vessels which have become dilated and are too large to respond to an electric needle may be treated through injection of a salt water solution. This skin problem, called cutaneous telangiectasia of the lower legs, may develop on any part of the leg, as well as on the ankles and feet. The injection of salt water has been used effectively to dry out and destroy the cells which make up the blood vessels. This procedure effectively eliminates the purplish lines which are outwardly visible, but does not prevent the formation of additional lines at a later date. Side effects are usually minimal, although in some cases bruising or blistering may develop. In rare cases, a blood clot may develop at the site, but it is not considered dangerous.

RETINOIDS

Vitamin A derivatives such as Retin-A and Accutane are being used to successfully control acne. Retin-A is a brand name for Vitamin A acid and is applied topically. As discussed in Chapter 7 (under Acne), this formula has the ability to destroy skin cells which clog follicles and facilitates the drying and peeling of dead skin cells that plug up the pores. Retin-A is available by prescription and involves a treatment period of several weeks to months before the usually excellent results appear. During the treatment process, the acne will often get worse before it gets better, and excessive dryness may occur. The results in most cases are worth the endurance. Accutane is another retinoid, taken internally and used for the management of severe acne.

Studies have indicated that certain retinoids may help repair collagen that has been damaged through sun exposure. Currently, the use of retinoids as anti-aging formulas is being explored. Some tests have shown that retinoids may retard to some degree the development of fine wrinkles and may promote the production of collagen in the dermal layer.

BENZOYL PEROXIDE

As discussed in Chapter 7, benzoyl peroxide is being applied successfully to treat all grades of acne. However, many preparations (both over-the-counter and by prescription) are available, and they vary in effectiveness. The formula to be used depends on the skin's condition, among other things.

The future for improving skin problems through dermatological treatments looks especially bright. Right now the techniques reviewed in this chapter are being used very successfully to upgrade the appearance of aging skin, to clear up acne, to remove solar keratoses and liverspots and to reduce the unsightly appearance of broken capillaries.

It is now clear that successful long-term management of healthy skin involves not just a narrow focus on the skin itself, but demands a sophisticated understanding and application of knowledge from many fields, including psychology, nutrition, biochemistry, genetics, and even environmental sciences. Early aging and serious skin disorders can often be prevented through an integrated self-care program that includes attention to *all* of the areas discussed in this book. The earlier in life this personalized program begins, the more rewarding will be the results.

9. Minding your Make-up

Make-up can serve as a great facial enhancer or it can detract from your skin's natural beauty. Its effect on your skin's health and appearance depends on your level of skill in make-up selection and application.

Self-knowledge is the first step toward effective use of make-up and other cosmetics. So, for starters, pull your hair back and away from the face. Then, using a hand mirror and a larger mirror, analyze your face from all angles. Study it up close and at a distance. Again, assess your basic skin type — oily, dry, normal, or combination. And identify the shape of your face — round, heart-shaped, oval, long or square. Once you understand your skin type and shape, move on to the details of your facial features. Do you have small eyes or large eyes, thin lips or full ones, thick or thin eyebrows? Is your nose narrow, wide, pudgy, or long? After taking note of your features you'll be ready to enhance them through skillful application of eye make-up, lipstick, foundation, blushers, and highlighters.

❧ SELECTION BASED ON SKIN TYPE

Selecting the right products for your skin and achieving the right look will naturally involve experimentation as well as feedback from friends or family. To begin, be sure face is cleansed and moisturized. If you apply a pre-make-up moisturizer, let it dissolve into the skin for a few minutes before going on with the make-up foundation. Check the following skin-type make-up selector chart to ensure that you are choosing products compatible with your skin type.

SKIN TYPE	*MAKE-UP TO SELECT*

Normal   Those with normal skin can use all types of make-up —both oily and non-oily preparations. It's still extremely important, however, that you choose your cosmetics with care. To protect and enhance your skin, you should become familiar with common cosmetic ingredients and then shop for quality products that will enhance your face without irritating it. For medium coverage, choose a liquid make-up. For light coverage, go with sheer or translucent make-up bases.

Oily   If your skin is oily, you need a water-based foundation that will control the outward appearance of oily skin. Avoid products containing large amounts of oil such as pancake foundations, and creamy foundations and blushers. Select a liquid foundation that is oil-free, brush-on blusher and eye shadow. Your lipstick should be light and contain a minimum of oil.

Dry   Dry skin needs to be protected with cream and oil-based products. Choose a day cream which helps moisturize and protect your skin and that allows your make-up foundation to glide on easily and evenly. A light, oil-based liquid or cream foundation will provide the best coverage for dry skin. Along the same line, choose creamy blushers, lipsticks, and eye make-up. Stay away from powder (which tends to dry out the skin); frosted cosmetics (which usually contain drying substances); and pancake make-up (which does not spread well on dry skin and serves to dry it even further). In selecting a foundation, keep in mind that you need a nice, creamy liquid that goes on easily and provides a heavier than average coverage.

❧ *FOUNDATIONS FOR FACIAL ENHANCEMENT*

The foundation you choose can make or break the outcome of your entire make-up job. The right product must not only be suited to your skin type, but it should be compatible with your skin's color, texture, and basic condition. A foundation can be sheer and light for clear, unblemished skin or it might be heavier to conceal blemishes or uneven pigmentation.

By day, you should apply a foundation close to your natural skin color. For evening wear, a shade darker can be enhancing, especially during the summer months. To locate the best choice of foundations, you'll have to experiment for awhile. If you know your skin well, understand basic make-up artistry, and the business of cosmetic manufacturing — you'll save much time and expense, as well as possible short-term or long-term damage to your skin.

Step 1: Day Cream

A protective, moisturizing day cream is vital for dry skin, is good for most types of normal skin, and should be used on aging skin to help counteract the normal drying process. Day cream is also called pre-make-up cream.

Step 2: Foundation

As indicated in the make-up selector chart, foundations should be chosen according to skin type and texture, skin color, and season. There are many types of foundations with many cosmetic lines carrying oil-free products for oily skin, rich, creamy products for dry skin, and special hypo-allergic products for sensitive skin. Such specialty products are not necessarily the best choice. Often, a regular cosmetic with the right combination of ingredients and usually less expensive, will turn out to be the most suitable and flattering to your skin. To decide, you'll need to read the labels and compare and experiment with the quality of the cosmetics. The list below provides a brief rundown on the basic types of foundations that are available.

Liquid Foundations

These come prepared for all skin types. There are oil-based formulas for normal and dry skin and oil-free products for oily skin. Generally, liquid bases provide a lighter coverage, although there are a few good liquids that provide excellent medium coverage. However, for corrective, concealing purposes, liquid foundations do not fare as well as other types.

Cream Foundations

These foundations may come in a jar, tube, or stick. Creams usually contain a larger amount of oil and are especially effective on dry skin. They are also useful for concealing facial blemishes or other disfigurations. For a flattering appearance, the cream must be applied evenly and consistently across the skin.

Pancake Foundation

This type of make-up provides heavy coverage and is extremely drying to the skin. Hence, it is best used on oily skin. However, there are other types of foundations that are more useful, even for oily skin. Pancake make-up has become a product of the past.

Gel Foundations

Gel make-up is good for normal skin and is especially popular during the summer when faces are tanned and less foundation is desired. The effect of a gel foundation is sheer, natural, and translucent and it is most useful in providing a minimum of coverage for unblemished skin.

Medicated Foundations

This type of make-up is designed for problem, blemished skin. Generally, medicated cosmetics are non-oily formulas that provide light to medium coverage and aid in drying up blemishes.

Hypo-allergenic Foundations

Hypo-allergenic make-up is helpful for very sensitive skin. Those with thin skin and who that are allergic to ingredients found in regular cosmetics may benefit from this type of special foundation.

Matte Foundation

Matte make-up bases combine both cream and powder. The formula is a good cover up and may be used on normal and oily skin, and on skin that is just slightly dry.

After comparing your skin type to the various foundations, you'll want to test for the right color. The best way to do this is to match your foundation color to the skin on your neck.

Now that you've selected both a suitable product and a flattering shade, you'll need to practice application. Start by dotting foundation on your cheeks, forehead, and chin. Blend in one side with a sweeping upward motion. Move to the other side and take care around the jawline, eyes, and nose. Wipe around the jawline to clear off any excess make-up and make sure you've applied the base evenly over the entire face. A make-up sponge may be used instead of fingertips.

❧ MAXIMIZING YOUR FACIAL FEATURES WITH FOUNDATION

Most foundations are not effective in hiding redness or dark circles under the eyes, irritation around the nose, or other types of skin problems. If you need to conceal a particular problem, choose a special cover stick or a liquid base that blends well with your skin tone. A green undercoat is used to conceal a ruddy complexion. If your skin is sallow or washed out, you can try a slightly pink shade for color enhancement. Or you can mix colors of the same line and produce your own unique shade. If your nose is long, minimize the flaw by blending a darker shade under the nasal base. Apply a darker shade along the sides to decrease the effect of a wide nose.

Around the nose and mouth area, use the cover stick to conceal lines. In essence, remember that a darker color decreases the effect of a feature, while light colors highlight the area. Go easy with foundation and concealer stick. Two coats of foundation is often most effective, especially for dry skin. But let the first coat sink in before applying the second. And don't overapply. It will only result in a caked appearance and will undermine whatever additional skill and effort you apply in finishing the make-up.

Blushing Beauty

As with foundation, blushers should be compatible with your skin color and type. The purpose of blushers is to contour, highlight, and add color to your complexion.

- *Cream blushers* are best applied after the make-up foundation. They contain oils and moisturizing agents and are designed for dry and normal skins. For the most effective application, wet your fingertips just slightly, dip into the blush and blend into the cheek area. Or use a damp make-up sponge.

- *Powder blushers* should be applied after the cream blush or after a slight dusting of powder depending on what works best for you. The use of powder is not recommended on very dry skin, but a small amount can be used effectively on combination skin and skin that is slightly dry.

- *Gel blushers* can be applied over a foundation or directly to the skin. This type of blusher is especially good during the summer suntan season and should be used without any powdering. Gels are usually found in a tube.

If your skin is oily, you need a powdered blush to control the oil, to highlight, and prevent make-up from fading and wearing off too soon. For dry skin, the best blush is a cream blush or one that is oil-based. And if your skin is normal, both powder or cream blushes can be enhancing. For all skin types, fading of make-up can often be a problem. One way to keep your make-up on longer is to apply a cream blush and then dust lightly with a powder blush. Blushers should be applied from the cheek bone outward. Depending on the shape of your face, you can blend the blusher in various ways to achieve your desired effect. The Facial Shape/Blusher chart that follows will help you apply blushers in a way that will best highlight your face.

☙ *FACIAL SHAPE/BLUSHER CHART*

Round

If your face is especially round, perhaps fat, or with a pudgy appearance, you need to minimize this effect while also creating the illusion of a high cheekbone. You can use a combination of pink and brown tones, with the brown being applied slightly under the cheekbones and shaded outward toward the ear area. While the brown base can provide some contouring and structuring to the face, a pink tone on top of the cheekbones can attractively highlight your face. Blend the pink blush in an outward motion toward the temple area. Another way is to apply blush on your cheekbones, starting in the center of your eyes and shading out and up toward the temples. Be sure the blush is well-blended so as not to leave any obvious line. The idea is to make it look as natural as possible.

Heart-Shape

Use any color that matches your skin. Blend in color from middle of cheekbone outward and down below ears a bit. Stay away from applying blusher on inner cheeks and too high into the temple area.

Long

To minimize the length of your face and create an illusion of more width, apply blush high on cheekbones and blend outward toward the hairline.

Square

An angular-type face can be de-emphasized by applying a shader below the cheekbones and down toward the jawline. Blend well to soften hard lines and traces of application. Apply blusher on upper cheeks above the shader and smooth it toward the temple area.

Oval

Smooth on blusher from cheekbones outward to the hairline. For variation, you can blend toward the temple area or apply blush lower on cheeks and blend up and away from the cheeks.

POWDER PRINCIPLES

A slight dusting of powder can set the make-up and is best used on normal and oily skin. A sheer or translucent type is a good choice as it looks natural and is not so heavy that it hides your make-up foundation and blush. A powder is not always necessary. A powdered blush over a cream blush also sets the make-up. If powder is used, it should be applied gently and sparingly.

EMPHASIZING EYES

Eyes should be made up to complement your face, to express your mood, and to reflect the natural beauty of your personality. Since the eyes need special attention and care, mastering the art of eye make-up application may take more time than other aspects of make-up. The basic steps in eye make-up include focusing on the brows, eye shadow, eye liner, and mascara. You may want to focus on one or all of these steps depending on the image you need to project.

Brows

Keep brows attractively tweezed and shaped. But go easy on the tweezing. Very thin brows are not only unattractive, they usually require more penciling which can appear artificial and detract from your basic beauty. Thick and well-shaped brows add an extra dimension of facial enhancement for many women. To find out whether you are more suited for thicker or thinner brows, experiment a bit. You should choose an eye brow pencil that is the same color as your brows and pencil in with short strokes, The idea is to keep them natural looking.

Eye Shadows

Eye shadows are used to emphasize the eyes, to enhance their color and size. Pale colors should be applied to highlight and increase eye prominence, while dark colors recede and decrease prominence. Eyes can be made to look smaller or larger, more prominent or less prominent and so on. Eye shadows, highlighters, and eyeliners will all contribute to the effect you want to create. For example, small eyes can be made-up to appear larger. Try a pale eyelid shade and then smudge a dark color in the crease. Be sure to blend in well to eliminate any hard lines. Use a dark eyeliner on the top of the eye, starting the line from the far corner and lining inward toward the nose. Line only half-way. At the base of the lash, line three quarters of the way from outer to inner corner of the eyes and then smudge a bit. Apply mascara on upper and lower lashes.

Eye shadows come in creams (oil-based and easy to smooth on); gels (easy to apply and long-lasting, but do not smooth easily into crease area); liquid shadows (available in wand or bottle, long-lasting, but harder to apply); powder shadows (applied with a sponge-tipped applicator or small brush, long-lasting). Since most eye shadows are long-lasting and available in numerous colors, your choice should depend on what works best for you.

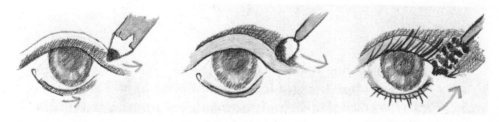

Eyeliner

Eyeliner is used for emphasis and may be applied in different ways depending on the effect you desire. Although liquid liner is widely used, a pencil is recommended. The eye area is particularly sensitive and should be protected. And although pencil liners may irritate the eyes, a liquid has greater potential to do so. In applying liquid liner it's much easier to slip and let liner seep into the eye area. In addition, even after the liquid liner dries, it tends to crack and flake which may ultimately harm the eyes. In choosing an appropriate eye pencil, look for a medium consistency. Hard pencils lack color and soft ones smudge — so shop until you find a good texture.

Mascara

Waterproof mascara is your best choice. Always apply two coats, but be sure the first coat is dry before attempting the second. Avoid over-application and products that clump lashes or weaken them. Again, you may have to try out a few different ones to find your ideal choice.

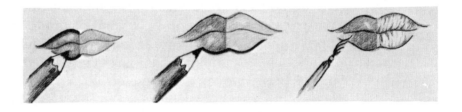

❧ *LIPS*

Thin lips: line your lip color a bit above and below the lipline.
Too-full lips: line just below the upper and lower lipline.
Dry or cracked lips: Apply petrolatum or lip gloss before lipstick to diminish the cracks. Use lip brush for best results.
Your best choice of color for foundation, blushers, eyeshadows, and lipsticks is related to your hair color and complexion. To get a better idea of which make-up colors to select, refer to the Make-up Color Chart that follows on page 121.

❧ *ENHANCING THE SKIN'S APPEARANCE THROUGH COLOR COORDINATION*

As advertising and marketing experts have long realized, color is an essential part of packaging — whether the package be a manufactured product or a human being. In selling products, color is a powerful part of the package that can turn a potential buyer from one product to another. It happens all the time in supermarkets and shopping centers when we are bombarded with color combinations — we flock to those items that are packaged attractively. In the human arena it may sound repugnant to talk of packaging based on colors, but the concept is the same. Our physical appearance — of which color is a part — represents our package. And this packaging tells the world a great deal about ourselves. It is not only an outward manifestation of our moods and emotions, but also an indicator of our personality, the image we have of ourselves, and the image we wish to project. To utilize color effectively, you must first understand its meaning. Only then can you be sure that you are using it to your advantage.

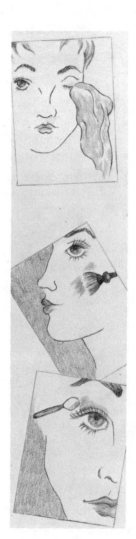

Choosing appropriate make-up colors to enhance skin and hair tones is but one part of the color process. Another step is putting together a wardrobe that reflects personality and complements one's skin and hair color.

Although there are people who look charming in just about any color style combination, most of us can benefit a great deal from a bit of color analysis. To learn about color and the ones that suit you best, you might want to attend a personal color workshop, request a private consultation, or even purchase a good book on color and do your own analysis. Since color is not a science, you won't find any right or wrong answers. In fact, the answers you do get will depend upon who is doing the analysis or which book you are reading. Different colors consultants may arrive at different conclusions about what your best colors are. (By the way, there are many well-trained color consultants around — probably some within your own area. However, you should do a little shopping and fact-finding before selecting a consultant.) Many consultants charge very reasonable fees, but some have set rather outrageous prices for the work that they actually do. As in other fields, there are those practitioners who are virtually untrained and have little interest in anything outside of money-making opportunities. After locating your method of color analysis, you should enter your period of study with an open mind. Then take the best of what you learn and formulate your own final ideas as to which shades and tones highlight your overall image.

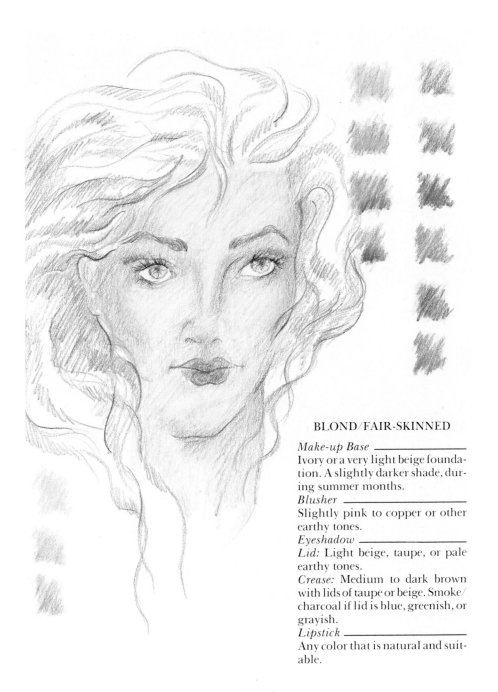

BLOND/FAIR-SKINNED

Make-up Base —————————
Ivory or a very light beige foundation. A slightly darker shade, during summer months.

Blusher —————————
Slightly pink to copper or other
earthy tones.

Eyeshadow —————————
Lid: Light beige, taupe, or pale
earthy tones.
Crease: Medium to dark brown
with lids of taupe or beige. Smoke/
charcoal if lid is blue, greenish, or
grayish.

Lipstick —————————
Any color that is natural and suitable.

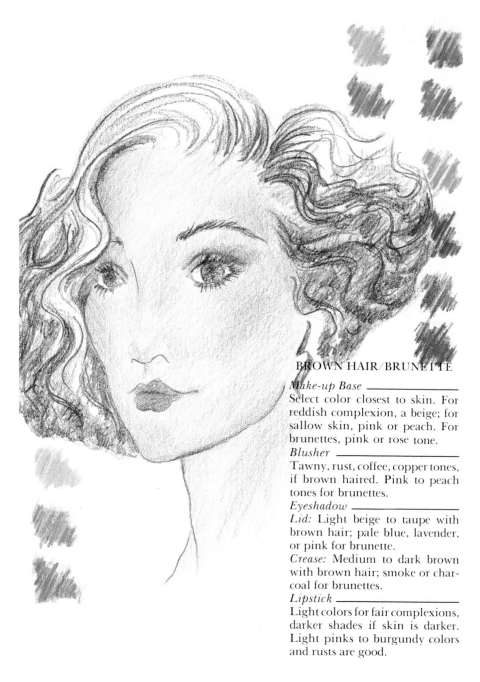

BROWN HAIR/BRUNETTE

Make-up Base ——————
Select color closest to skin. For reddish complexion, a beige; for sallow skin, pink or peach. For brunettes, pink or rose tone.

Blusher ——————
Tawny, rust, coffee, copper tones, if brown haired. Pink to peach tones for brunettes.

Eyeshadow ——————
Lid: Light beige to taupe with brown hair; pale blue, lavender, or pink for brunette.
Crease: Medium to dark brown with brown hair; smoke or charcoal for brunettes.

Lipstick ——————
Light colors for fair complexions, darker shades if skin is darker. Light pinks to burgundy colors and rusts are good.

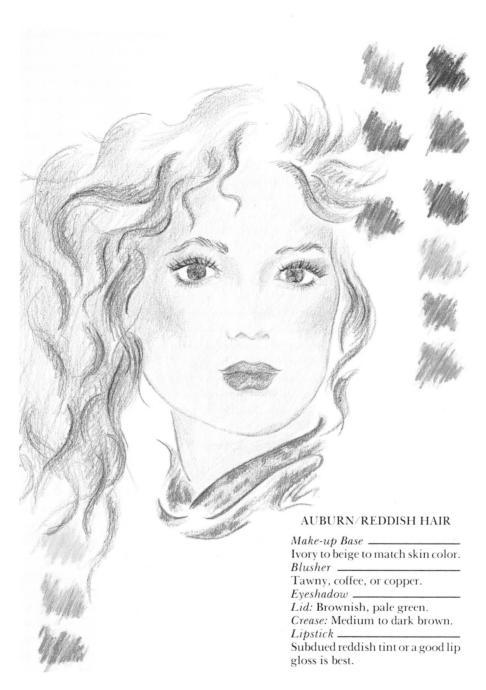

AUBURN/REDDISH HAIR

Make-up Base _____
Ivory to beige to match skin color.
Blusher _____
Tawny, coffee, or copper.
Eyeshadow _____
Lid: Brownish, pale green.
Crease: Medium to dark brown.
Lipstick _____
Subdued reddish tint or a good lip
gloss is best.

[123]

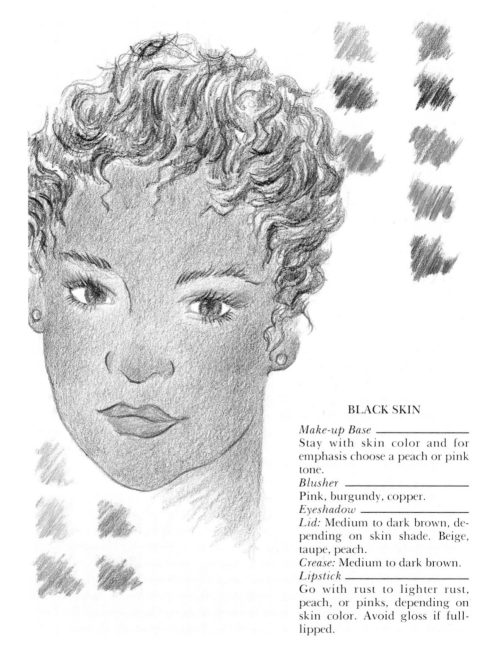

BLACK SKIN

Make-up Base ———————
Stay with skin color and for emphasis choose a peach or pink tone.

Blusher ———————
Pink, burgundy, copper.

Eyeshadow ———————
Lid: Medium to dark brown, depending on skin shade. Beige, taupe, peach.
Crease: Medium to dark brown.

Lipstick ———————
Go with rust to lighter rust, peach, or pinks, depending on skin color. Avoid gloss if full-lipped.

[124]

10. Protecting and Treating your Skin

✤ DEEP CLEANSING VIA STEAM

To reap the rewards of a home-made gentle steam bath, boil some water and find a comfortable place to sit down with a towel covering your head. Dip your face into the steam, keeping it about a foot or so away from the water.

The steam will open up clogged areas, loosening built-up facial debris. After steaming, rinse with tepid water and apply a sloughing treatment to smooth the skin and remove any remaining surface grime. For variety in your steaming regimen, add one of the following herbal solutions to the water.

To prepare your herbal steam mixture, add 2-3 tablespoons of an herb or combination of herbs to a pot of boiling water. Be sure and select herbs suitable for your skin type.

Some Herbs for Oily Skin

Anise	Lavender	Papaya
Apricot	Lemon	Rose
Fennel	Licorice	Witch Hazel

Some Herbs for Dry Skin

Acacia	Comfrey Root	Licorice
Aloe Vera	Honeydew	Mint
Chamomile	Irish Moss	Orange Blossom

[125]

Dry to Normal Skin

Licorice	Comfrey Root
Fennel	Chamomile
Clover	

Oily to Normal Skin

Witch Hazel	Lemongrass
Roses	Lavender
Lemon Peel	

⚜ SAUNAS

Saunas have the same impact on skin as do steam treatments. The moist heat not only stimulates circulation, but helps unclog the pores and loosen dead skin that needs to be exfoliated for a smoother appearance.

⚜ FACIALS

Often the best facials are the ones that you give yourself. If you care about your skin, then you'll be gentle with it — most likely giving it more tender loving care than would a professional esthetician. But a word about self-administered facials. When you do a facial on yourself, you'll be applying some type of solution or masque to your skin. What you need to remember is that the face normally gets enough manipulating through make-up application and removal, creaming, sloughing, and so forth. So you need to be extra careful to massage your skin gently and briefly. Pimples, if necessary, should be extracted professionally. Also, be aware of what ingredients you're applying to your face. Another reminder: just because an avocado and sesame oil mish mash is good for your friend's face doesn't mean it will help yours. Get informed about your skin's needs and the best products that can fulfill those needs. Stay away from fads and constant application of mixed ingredients. Just as good health cannot be bought at the drugstore, neither will healthy skin grow out of a cosmetic jar.

Masques may be gel (an aid for dry skin) or clay (noted for oily skin). Masques may also be granular with a base of oatmeal, cornmeal, or almonds. Other masques may be primarily oil-based. In essence, there are many kinds of masques and semi-facial treatments for every conceivable skin type. There are masques that aid blemishes, those that tighten, rejuvenate, refresh, smooth and tone the skin. You'll also find formulas that will temporarily reduce the appearance of bags and wrinkles. These products certainly do not provide any real protection against aging nor do they have any permanent results. Although they may contain ingredients known to lessen the production or appearance of wrinkles, (collagen, for example) such products are not effective when applied topically because they cannot be properly absorbed. In the case of collagen, positive results are sometimes seen when the collagen is injected directly into the skin.

Facial Masque Application

Before applying any masque the face should be cleansed thoroughly. Clean as usual, then steam clean and apply one of your favorite masques. After the masque has set for 10-15 minutes or longer, rinse with warm, then cool water.

⚜ MASQUES FOR ALL SKIN TYPES

Buttermilk Masque

⅓ cup of rolled oats soaked several hours in buttermilk. Strain. Add 1 capsule of Vitamin A (10,000 IU) and mix well. After cleansing skin, apply mixture and leave on 10-15 minutes. Rinse with tepid water.

Flour Masque

⅓ cup of whole wheat flour mixed with enough milk to form a paste. Apply to face and leave on 15-20 minutes. Remove with warm water. Store excess for a maximum of three days in refrigerator.

Almond Meal Masque

Grind 25 almonds or buy ready-to-use almond meal. Mix almond meal with a slice of peeled aloe. Add a few drops of sesame oil and mix together until blended. Dampen face slightly with a bit of milk or warm water. Apply masque and leave on for 15 minutes. Then rinse with warm water.

Orange Cornmeal Delight

Take one peeled orange and put in blender along with your desired amount of cornmeal. Add ¼ cup uncooked oatmeal and mix well. Apply to a slightly damp face. Leave on for 10 minutes, then spray a bit of warm water on face and use circular motion to work masque around face. Remove with warm water.

Yogurt and Honey Masque

Mix together 1 teaspoon honey, 1 capsule of Vitamin A (10,000 IU), 1 tablespoon yogurt and ¾ egg yolk. To thicken, add a small amount of cornstarch. Apply masque to clean skin and leave on for 20 minutes. Rinse with lukewarm water.

Oatmeal-Honey Masque

   ½ cup uncooked oatmeal
   3 tablespoons honey
   1 egg yolk

Mix all ingredients together and apply over entire face. Rub masque around face in circular motion. Leave on for 10 minutes.

Natural Mineral Water Masque

Select a quality mineral water and pour into plastic spray bottle. Rich in magnesium (a moisture-retention agent) and other important minerals, this mist should be used to moisturize and refresh the face, to set make-up, soothe skin problems, and maintain freshness during exercise or sports-related activities.

Creamy Avocado and Honey Masque

   2 tablespoons avocado, mashed
   3 tablespoons honey
   1 whole egg

Whip until smooth and creamy in blender. Apply to entire face and leave on 10-15 minutes. This formula serves to tighten (eggs encourage the tightening sensation), and smooth the skin. Since it becomes hard after application, you'll need to remove with warm water.

Skin Nourishing Masque

   2 tablespoons honey
   3 tablespoons olive or mineral oil
   1 whole egg

Mix together egg yolk, oil and honey. Stir thoroughly. Now add egg white. Close container and shake well before applying.

Formula F Plus

   In the book, *Swedish Beauty Secrets,* Dr. Paavo Airola prescribes the following mixture as a natural skin treatment.*

   2 tablespoons sesame oil
   1 tablespoon olive oil
   2 tablespoons avocado oil
   1 tablespoon almond oil
   2,000 I.U. Vitamin E
   100,000 USP units Vitamin A
   a drop of your favorite perfume

Mix all ingredients in a small bottle or jar. Close the cap tightly and shake well. Store in refrigerator.

----

* Paavo A. Airola, *Swedish Beauty Secrets* (Phoenix, AZ: Health Plus Publishers, 1982), pp. 24-25

Besan* and Milk Masque

Mix H cup besan flour with enough milk to make a paste. Refrigerate for a few hours and apply over entire face. Leave on 15-20 minutes. Since the masque becomes hard, use warm water to rinse off. Then splash on cool water. An effective skin tightening mix, this masque serves as a deep-cleansing agent, removing both surface grime and other skin impurities.

* Besan flour may be purchased as gram flour in Asian specialty markets.

❧ MASQUES FOR OILY SKIN

Mashed Cucumber Masque

Mix mashed cucumber with oatmeal or almond meal. Add 1 tablespoon avocado oil and enough lemon juice to form a paste. Apply to clean skin and leave on for 15-20 minutes.

Facial Refining Masque

Mix ⅓ cup Kaolin (China Clay) with ¼ cup cornstarch. Add ¾ teaspoon of alum and enough olive oil to make a workable paste. This mixture serves as a skin tightener and becomes rather hard when applied to the skin. You may substitute egg white for oil and achieve the same tightening effect. For easiest removal, use warm water.

Banana and Brewer's Yeast

Mash one peeled banana. Add desired amount of brewer's yeast and milk. Blend ingredients well and apply thickened mixture to face, leaving on 15 minutes. Rinse with warm water and apply an astringent.

Strawberry Apricot Cool

Steam face with your favorite herbal mix. Remove a few cool strawberries from container (without excess juice). Mash and mix with powdered apricot. Add almond meal and a bit of comfrey root. Mix ingredients to form desired thickness. Leave on for 15 minutes and remove with warm water.

✌ *MASQUES FOR DRY SKIN*

Nourishing Dry Skin Facial

3 tablespoons olive oil
1 egg yolk
1 avocado, well mashed
1 Vitamin A capsule (10,000 I.U.)
1 tablespoon powdered Irish Moss

Petrolatum

To soften dry skin, simply apply a generous amount of petrolatum to face and leave on for at least one-half hour.

Mayonnaise Masque

Mix ⅓ cup mayonnaise with a few drops of milk. Add enough almond meal to make a paste. Apply to skin and let it stay on for 15-20 minutes.

The "Scandinavian Freeze"

Mix together 1 cup mineral water, ½ cup freshener, and a sprinkling of powdered alum. Poor mixture into ice cube tray, filling each cube about ¾ full. Place a popsicle stick or similar stick into each cube. Later, when water freezes, you can pop up one cube and with the stick as your handle, smooth over your face. To firm and tighten the skin and temporarily lessen the appearance of sags and wrinkles, press the ice cube over the problem areas.

❧ *A SAMPLING OF HOME-MADE SKIN TREATMENTS*

Cream of Rosewater (for Dry Skin)

2 tablespoons glycerin

3 ounces sesame oil*

¾ - ½ ounce beeswax

¼ ounce almond oil

¾ ounce rosewater

1 capsule of Vitamin A (10,000 I.U.)

Melt beeswax in top of double boiler. While stirring constantly, add each oil, glycerin and Vitamin A. Reduce to simmer and add rosewater. Continue stirring until mixture has cooled. Pour into jar and label with notation of contents.

   * NOTE: Sesame oil should be used with care as it may act as a skin irritant.

Cream of Strawberry (for Oily Skin)

2 tablespoons powdered apricot

2 ounces strawberry juice

2 ounces cocoa butter

2 ounces sweet almond oil

2 tablespoons lemon juice

Melt cocoa butter in double boiler. Blend in almond oil and powdered apricot. Remove from heat. Add strawberry juice and whip together as mixture cools. Sprinkle with 2 tablespoons lemon juice and whip again until mixture is well-blended and cooled. After application, rinse with cool water.

Alum Astringent (for Dry Skin)

8 ounces mineral water

¾ teaspoon aluminum salt

Mix well, label, and store in refrigerator. Discard after two months.

Home-Made Eye Cream

½ ounce cocoa butter
¾ ounce lanolin
½ ounce olive oil
½ ounce avocado oil
¼ ounce soy oil
3,000 I.U. of Vitamin E (Capsules can be punctured and squeezed into mixture)

Melt lanolin and cocoa butter in double boiler and add the oils, one at a time. Stir and blend well, pour into labeled container. Before sleep, apply mixture to eye area and use consistently.

Granular Scrub (for Blemished or any Type Skin)

Select your favorite meal — oatmeal, cornmeal, or almond meal, and mix in a bit of yogurt or milk (regular or buttermilk). Apply to face and use circular motion to scrub. Use 3-4 times a week. For more stimulation, use a loofah (Buff-Puff type sponge) to scrub your face with this mixture.

Fruit and Vegetable Peel

Facial peeling, often referred to as exfoliation, can also be achieved by applying the mashed pulp of avocado, lemon, orange or other fruit/veggies of your choice.

Chapped Lips Formula

Melt 3 ounces beeswax with 1 tablespoon of camphor, 3 ounces of sesame oil and 2 tablespoons of glycerin. Add 1 capsule of Vitamin E (1,000 I.U.). Pure petrolatum jelly is another effective formula for treatment of chapped lips.

Throat Cream

Mix 2 tablespoons of mashed avocado with a small amount of anhydrous lanolin. Apply to throat area and massage.

Vitamin E can also be used as a nourishing aid for the throat.

Herbal Steam Treatment (for Acne)

3 tablespoons comfrey leaf

2 tablespoons dandelion

2 tablespoons fennel seed

3 tablespoons licorice root

2 ounces white willow bark

Mix into boiling water and follow normal steaming procedure.

Facial Treatment for Clogged Pores

To promote eradication of blackheads, it's important to keep the skin soft. Herbal waters such as comfrey, fennel seed, or marshmallow root may be used to aid in unclogging pores. Simply add 2-3 tablespoons of your chosen herb to a pot of boiling water and then reduce to simmer. After the mixture has cooled, apply to face with cottonball. May be repeated several times a day. Herbal waters should be prepared fresh with daily use. Hot herbal compresses can be very helpful in clearing out blackheads. Saturate a soft cloth with hot herbal water and pat face for a few minutes.

To refine and texturize a skin that is filled with clogged pores, meals such as cornmeal, almond meal, or barley meal can be mixed with water, milk or yogurt and applied in a circular motion to face.

❧ HERBAL BODY TREATMENT FOR TOTAL SKIN MAINTENANCE

Healthy skin results through control of many factors such as good dietary habits, regular exercise, and avoidance of prolonged stress. Cleanliness, use of suitable skin care products, and minimal contact with harsh environmental elements are also vitally important to skin maintenance. The skin is not only the most exposed bodily organ, but it's also the largest. It consists of two layers — the dermis and the epidermis. The top layer is the epidermis and is composed of cells that divide to form new cells. The new cells, which rise to the surface of the epidermis, harden and become a type of protein called keratin. The dead protein layer can be peeled off by exfoliation.

Should it remain on the surface of the skin, it combines with oil and bacteria and develops into body odor. Below the epidermis is the dermis which is made up of blood vessels, hair roots, nerve endings, and glands that produce sebum and sweat. And below these structures is fat. Between these three layers are the muscle fibers and connective tissue that bind it all together and ensure that the skin structure is strong and healthy.

Now, there are as many overall body treatment shampoos as there are facial formulas. The herbal bath is one way to condition the entire skin. Since there are so many possible bath formulas, you'll have to experiment and find your own favorite. But to get you started, a few suggestions are listed below.

Skin Bath Delight

Try combining 1 ounce each of the following herbs: dried roses, aloe, lavender, peppermint, and comfrey root.

Herbal Bath

Mix 1 ounce each of lavender, wintersweet, roses, and violet leaves. Add your favorite essence and enjoy the results.

Saltwater Shampoo #2

Mix ½ pound of sea salt, ¼ pound powdered Irish moss, 2 ounces comfrey root, ¼ pound bicarbonate of soda. Add oil of mink and pour desired amount into your bath for a refreshing body shampoo.

⚘ BATH OILS

Bath oils can be effective in the treatment of dry skin and related skin problems. Often dry skin develops because of poor nutrition, environmental elements, changes in metabolism, or other factors. Regular use of natural bath oil can aid in the relief of dry and scaling skin, chapped and itching skin, dermatitis, psoriasis, and similar skin disorders. Basically, a bath oil applied to the body soothes the outer skin and prevents against additional loss of moisture.

In general, there are two categories of bath oil — floating oils and those that disperse in water. Floating oils may leave a ring around the tub, while dispersible oil dissolves into the water and usually leaves no ring. Both types of oil can be beneficial in minimizing some skin discomforts and in soothing and smoothing the skin. Selecting a bath oil, then, is a matter of preference. And there are certainly many types which you can develop at home.

✤ FLOATING BATH OILS

Tropical Bath Oil

½ cup almond oil
¾ cup avocado oil
½ cup coconut oil (melted)
¼ cup safflower oil
¼ cup apricot kernel oil
¾ ounce lemon peel oil
¾ ounce orange peel oil
Mix together and shake well.

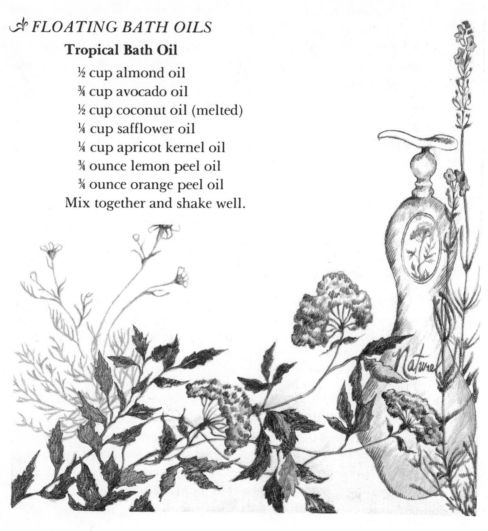

Oriental Spice Bath

¼ cup melted coconut oil
½ ounce Jasmine oil
¼ cup apricot kernel oil
½ ounce oil of lavender
¼ ounce oil of mink
¾ cup sesame seed oil
Mix together and shake well.

Flowered Bath Oil

½ cup almond oil
½ cup safflower oil
¾ ounce essential oil of rose
¼ cup essential oil of lavender
½ ounce honeysuckle oil
¼ cup sunflower oil
¼ cup olive oil
Mix together and shake well.

✣ WATER DISPERSIBLE OILS

Refreshing Rose Bath Oil

In a double boiler, melt ½ cup hydrous lanolin. Continue stirring and add 1 cup olive oil and ¾ cup wheat germ oil. Slowly pour in ¾ cup unscented alcohol that has been mixed with ¼ cup of essential oil of rose and ¼ cup essential oil of violets. Mix all ingredients together. Pour into bottle and shake well.

Along with bath oils come body oils. The main difference between the two is that body oils are usually less scented and are applied to the body via massage. If your skin is dry or even if it's normal, frequent use of after-bath body oils can provide an extra bonus for the skin. You will always want to use oils that are suitable for your skin type. Thus, the chart below is an example of common oils and their classifications.

Nondrying oils (for dry skin); usually come from tropical plants: olive, peanut, almond, cacao (cocoa butter), castor, palm.

Partially drying oils (for normal to oily skin): cottonseed, corn, sesame, sunflower.

Drying oils (for oily skin), for a better result, combine with other oils: soybean, tung, linseed, and many nut oils.

After total skin cleansing and conditioning, there is specific spot work to be done. Although each part of the skin is really a separate spot, (feet, hands, neck, back, legs, etc.), mention will be made here of only the hands and feet since these two areas are often in need of extra attention. To prevent against a dry, chapped, or well-worn appearance, give these parts extra special care. Again, you can make your own formulas or select effective commercial products.

Hand and Feet Softening Treatment

Combine 3 tablespoons oatmeal with 1 tablespoon honey, 1 egg yolk well beaten, and 2 tablespoons cocoa butter.

Basic Hand and Feet Formula

Mix sesame oil with softened honey and apply to hands and feet. Leave on overnight. Cover feet with socks, hands with gloves. Upon arising, soak in hot salt water.

Another formula to tone and smooth the skin is a mix of wheat oil, Vitamin E, and wheat germ oil. Leave on for one-half hour and rinse off.

Cocoa Butter Skin Softener

Both hands and feet can benefit from a mixture of cocoa butter and wheat germ oil. Apply mixture after bathing and using a pumice stone on problem areas.

11. Focusing on the Cosmetic Label

The cosmetic industry continues to be one of the largest advertisers and this is especially true for T.V. and magazine advertising. Such advertising can provide a valuable service to the public. It may introduce consumers to products and services that are useful and effective. And learning what is available in the market through advertising can also save time and may provide information that would otherwise be difficult to uncover. But there are also major drawbacks. Advertising often results in exaggerated claims being made about a product; the result is misleading information to the consumer. There is also such a vast array of cosmetic products available that it is almost impossible to choose the most appropriate and reasonably-priced product, without some specialized knowledge of the basic products and their ingredients.

Unless one is a chemist, the process of understanding labels and determining which products are most suitable can be a time-consuming and difficult task.

The aim of this chapter is to provide consumers with information that is practical and useful in determining the basic function and worth of a cosmetic product.

Cosmetics traditionally have received little attention from the regulatory level in the U.S. This has been true primarily because it was largely assumed that these products and techniques have little effect on individual health. Human skin was once considered practically impenetrable. The belief was that the skin shielded the body from the effects of chemicals applied to its outer surface.

[139]

During the 1960's, however, certain drugs such as DMSO were shown not only to penetrate the skin, but to carry along harmful substances into the body and bloodstream. Since that time new scientific investigations have continued to show the relationship between chemical applications to the skin and their effect on the body. As a result, FDA regulations regarding cosmetic manufacturing practices and labeling have also changed. Today monitoring of cosmetics is still by no means a top priority for the FDA. Some additional safety measures have been developed and implemented, but the bulk of cosmetic surveillance — if it is to be accomplished —must occur through individual concerns and consumer initiative.

Since 1976 all commercially-marketed cosmetic products must list ingredients. One exemption to this policy has included fragrances. As it now stands, all cosmetic products must list ingredients (by standardized names) in order of prevalence on the cosmetic label. This notice of ingredients may be found on the cosmetic box or on the label of the cosmetic product itself.

Although it is beyond the scope of this chapter, it is worth mentioning that many ingredients prohibited by other countries are allowed in American cosmetic products. A number of other nations also have more stringent registration, licensing, and production requirements than does the U.S. In Japan, for example, the use of ingredients such as mercury, hydroquinone, and dichlorophene is banned. And for a large number of other ingredients the Japanese government places restrictions on the quantity of the chemical that can be added to a product. In addition, the substance must meet government specifications and requirements. The labels not only must list ingredients by their standard name, but must indicate the amounts of such ingredients. Furthermore, cosmetic manufacturers are required to have government licenses. To receive a license, certain members of the industry are required to meet established eductional standards.

A common complaint about cosmetic products has to do with the allergic reactions or skin irritations that many people experience. Reactions always vary from individual to individual. But one thing is certain. The more chemicals applied to the skin, the greater the chance of adverse reactions. In conjunction with chemicals externally applied, there is the consumption of foods and drugs laden with chemicals that combine to increase the likelihood of a "cross-chemical" or "cross-sensitivity" reaction. In essence, this means that as the body is exposed to greater numbers of chemicals — both internally and externally — the chances of adverse reactions increase.

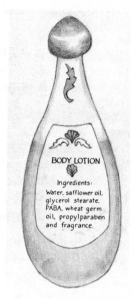

In recent years public outcry has resulted in the development of so-called "hypoallergenic" products. However, the consensus among government regulators and authorities in the field is that the term "hypoallergenic" does not live up to its intended meaning. Originally, the term was to mean "nonallergenic" products. But then it was realized that a nonallergenic product does not exist since there will always be some individual who is allergic to a certain substance. In light of the "hypoallergenic" definition problem, the FDA required that a number of ingredients be tested for allergic reactions. The plan was to remove or reduce the usage of those ingredients (in the test group) causing an adverse reaction in a significant number of exposed individuals. Then, with this measure of protection, a product could safely be called "hypoallergenic." In order to promote a product as "hypoallergenic" the FDA has set forth only certain minimum requirements and the issue is still being debated. Stricter policies have not materialized primarily because of disagreements over appropriate testing methods and because of problems surrounding enforcement of imposed standards. The FDA did, however, rule that once a company labels a product as "hypoallergenic," it has two and a half years to substantiate that claim. The subject continues to be a sensitive one and comprehensive, and uniform requirements have yet to be implemented.

A similar but less complicated problem involves the public demand for use of organic and natural products. Although natural or organic products have long been utilized in cosmetic formulas, they have not always been promoted as such. To keep pace with current health fads and consumer demands, "new" products have appeared on the market to satisfy the cry for more natural and organically based formulas. New labeling and fancy packaging in products has also resulted in price increases. Of course, as mentioned elsewhere in this book, price is not an indicator of quality. There are many products with similar or identical ingredients but with very different price tags. Cold creams, cleansing creams, and lipsticks are but a few examples. Other products such as petrolatum have been shown to serve the same purpose as the expensive and attractively packaged emollients. This is equally true of many vegetable oils which provide the same benefits as highly priced oils and moisturizers with updated labels and attractive packaging. Across the board, cosmetic manufacturers have continud to capitalize on the consumer-oriented notion that the higher the price, the better the results.

The purpose of the glossary that follows is to enable the reader to easily locate some of the most common cosmetic ingredients, cosmetic products and their classifications. By reading labels and comparing products based on their ingredients (rather than on price, packaging, or promotional techniques) the consumer is equipped to make more intelligent purchasing decisions. You will be able to evaluate a product more accurately, based on its ingredients and you will learn to evaluate advertising claims. (Do the products actually do what they say they will do?) Of equal importance, you will also save yourself a lot of time and money in selecting cosmetic products. And finally, you will know (on the basis of ingredients) which products to avoid or use sparingly.

Glossary

ACETIC ACID.
A transparent colorless liquid with a strong odor. Used in hand lotions, hair dyes, and freckle-bleaching formulas. Concentrations of even less than 5% may act as a mild skin irritant. Acetic acid combined with certain other substances is known as acetyl.

ACETYLATEDPALM KERNEL GLYCERIDES.
Oil extracted from the seed of the African palm. It is used in soaps and ointments.

ACID BALANCE.
This term means that the cosmetic product's pH is equivalent to the pH of the skin or hair.

ALBUMIN.
Used in astringents and facial masques to create the tight feeling and as an emulsifier in other cosmetics. For cosmetic use, albumin frequently comes from egg white.

ALCOHOL.
A solvent in many cosmetic products and used externally as an antiseptic. Very drying to the skin.

ALKALI.
pH greater than 7. Used as an acid neutralizer in cosmetics.

ALLANTOIN.
A colorless skin-soothing ingredient that is found in cold creams, hand lotions, and other cosmetics. Nontoxic.

[143]

ALLERGEN.
A substance that triggers an allergic reaction.

ALMOND MEAL.
Derived from blanched almonds, this powdery meal is used in cosmetics for its soothing qualities.

ALMOND OIL.
Found in many cosmetic products such as eye creams, emollients, and soaps. Known to cause skin rashes and nasal congestion in susceptible individuals.

ALOE VERA.
Taken from the aloe plant leaf, aloe vera is found in all kinds of cosmetic products. Advertised as a substance that softens and heals, but scientific evidence is lacking. When applied externally, it is non-toxic.

ALUM.
An ingredient widely used in astringents. Found in other products such as antiperspirants, fresheners, and after-shave lotions.

ALUMINUM POWDER.
A color additive in facial powders and hair colorings.

ALUMINUM STEARATE.
Used for coloring and thickening in cosmetics. No known toxicity.

ALUMINUM SULFATE.
A crystalline substance used as an antiseptic, astringent, and detergent in deodorants, skin fresheners, antiperspirants, and related products.

AMINOMETHYL PROPANEDIOL.
An emulsifier in cosmetic creams, lotions, and mineral oils.

AMMONIUM IODIDE.
Made from ammonia and iodine. In cosmetics it is used as an antiseptic and preservative.

ANESTHETIC.
A substance that produces partial or total loss of physical sensibility.

ANTISEPTIC.
Agent used to inhibit growth of bacteria (e.g. alcohol and hexachlorophene).

APRICOT.
Crushed apricot is used in facial masques to soften skin. Apricot oil may be used in some cosmetic creams.

ARACHIDONIC ACID.
An unsaturated fatty acid that is used to sooth skin rashes and eczema and is found in cosmetic creams and lotions.

ARNICA.
Used as an astringent and sometimes found in skin fresheners.

AROMATIC.
For cosmetic purposes, the term refers to chemicals having an aroma.

ASCORBIC ACID. (Vitamin C)
A preservative and antioxidant in various cosmetic creams. Non-toxic.

ASCORBYL PALMITATE.
A nontoxic preservative and antioxidant used in cosmetic creams and lotions. A salt derived from ascorbic acid that is used to prevent rancidity.

ASTRINGENT.
Promoted as a skin toning agent for oily skin. Usually high in alcohol. Should not be used on dry or very sensitive skin.

AVOCADO OIL.
Found in lubricating creams, shampoos, and masques. Nontoxic.

BALM MINT.
Used as an unguent (provides soothing effect on the skin) in cosmetics and may also be found in perfumes (as a fragrance).

BANANA.
Rich in potassium, this popular fruit is frequently used as an aid for dry skin and is found in home-made facial masques. Banana flavoring or artificial banana may be found in some cosmetics.

BATH OIL.
The purpose of bath oils is to soften, smooth, and protect the skin. Most such oils are highly fragranced and may be purchased in a foam or non-foam oil. Bath oils should be kept away from the eye area and may cause slight skin irritations in some cases.

BATH SALTS.
The aim of bath salts is to impart a fragrance to the skin, and to perfume and color bath water. Certain chemicals in bath salts help soften the water and may be soothing to the skin. Rock salt and sodium thiosulfate are common base ingredients. Many other chemicals are present in bath salts, and some of these (e.g. borax and phosphate) may irritate the skin.

BAYBERRY WAX.
Employed as an astringent in soaps and hair products. May irritate the skin.

BAY RUM.
An oil extracted from the leaves of bayberry and combined with rum or with alcohol, water, and additional oils. Used as a skin freshener. May cause allergic reaction.

BEESWAX.
Manufactured by bees and used primarily as an emulsifier in cosmetics. It is found in cold cream, emollient creams, eye creams, foundation creams and make-up, mascara, lipstick, rouge, and others.

BENTONITE.
White clay used as a thickener and emulsifier in masques and lotions.

BENZALDEHYDE. (Artificial almond oil)
Made from the kernels of bitter almonds, it is found in soaps, perfumes, creams and lotions. Can cause allergic reactions.

BENZOIN.
Found in protective creams, freckle and bleaching creams, skin fresheners, and lipstick, and used as a preservative in ointments. May cause allergic reactions.

BIOTIN.
Found in very small amounts in all living cells and also present in milk and yeast. A texturizer in cosmetic creams, biotin is a white powder necessary for human growth, healthy circulation and red blood cells.

BIRCH.
This substance has long been used as a treatment for rheumatism, as a laxative, and to relieve symptoms of gout. It is used in creams and shampoos as an astringent and has been known to aid in the healing of certain skin breakouts.

BLACKHEAD.
Open comedo. See "comedo."

BLUSHER.
Found in powder, cream, or stick form. Used primarily to provide color and to contour the cheeks.

BORATES.
In cosmetics it is used as an antiseptic, preservative, and texturizer. May be extremely toxic.

BORAX.
This is a mild alkali used as an emulsifier, preservative, and texturizer in some products. It is usually found in cold creams, foundation creams, cleansing lotions, and certain hair products.

BUTYLATED HYDROXYANISOLE. (BHA)
A white to pale yellow solid, used as a preservative and antioxidant in cosmetics. May cause allergic reactions.

BUTYLATED HYDROXYTOLUENE. (BHT)
A whitish crystalline solid, used as a preservative and antioxidant in cosmetics.

BUTYL STEARATE.
Widely used as an emulsifier. Found in creams, lipstick, bath products, and nail polish remover. May cause skin irritation.

CAFFEINE.
A whitish powder found naturally in cola, coffee, tea, guarana, and other products. The role of caffeine in cosmetic products has not been clearly established.

CALAMINE.
Found in astringents, lotions, ointments, protective creams and other cosmetic products designated for the treatment of skin diseases.

CALCIUM CARBONATE. (Chalk)
An odorless powder that is found in marble, limestone, and coral. It is used as a white coloring agent in cosmetics, as a neutralizer and firming agent, and is found in bleaches. It may be used as a buffer in face powders and is found in other cosmetics as well.

CALCIUM PANTOTHENATE. (Vitamin B₅)
An emollient in cosmetic creams and lotions. Nontoxic.

CAMPHOR.
Known for its cooling quality, camphor is used as an antiseptic and rubefactant. An aid for chapped and itchy skin. Absorbed through the skin and capable of causing skin rashes and allergic reactions.

CARAMEL.
Used in cosmetics as a coloring agent. Has a soothing quality and is found in skin lotions. Produced by heating glucose or sugar and adding small amounts of alkali or a trace mineral.

CARAWAY OIL.
From the ripe fruit, this oil carries the aroma of caraway and is used to perfume soap. Can cause skin irritations and allergic reactions.

CARBOMER.
A mildly acidic, white powder that combines with fatty substances to produce thick emulsions of oils in water. In cosmetic products, it is used primarily as a thickening agent and as an emulsifier.

CARBON DIOXIDE.
A noncombustible gas found in some creams. In cryotherapy, freezing with carbon dioxide (CO_2) is sometimes used to treat keratoses, although it has been largely replaced by liquid nitrogen.

CARNAUBA WAX.
Derived from the carnauba palm tree and used as a texturizer in cosmetics. This brown-colored wax is found in creams, deodorant sticks, and depilatory waxes.

CAROTENE.
In cosmetics, carotene is used as a coloring agent. It also provides a yellow color to carrots, egg yolks, and butter. It is nontoxic to the skin.

CARROT OIL.

Extracted from carrot seeds, this essential oil is pale yellow, has a spicy aroma, and is found in perfumes. May also be used as a coloring agent. It is not known to cause skin reactions.

CASTILE SOAP.

This hard soap is made from olive oil and sodium hydroxide. Named after the Spanish region where it was originally used, Castile soap is usually white, yellowish white, or green.

CASTOR OIL.

Derived from the castor bean, this oil has qualities similar to those found in most vegetable oils. Its odor is unpleasant, but it is found in some bath oils, nail polish removers, face masques, lipsticks, eye-drops, and others. Generally nontoxic when applied to the skin but may cause skin reaction in susceptible individuals.

CELLULOSE GUMS.

Includes a group of fibrous substances composed from the cell walls of plants. It may be used in lipstick (in the form of ethyl-cellulose) and as an emulsifier in hand creams and lotions (as methylcellulose or methocel and hydroxyethylcellulose or cellosize).

CETYL ALCOHOL.

An emollient and emulsion stabilizer in many cosmetics such as mascaras, cream rouges, and hand lotions. Known to have a low degree of toxicity for skin.

CHAMOMILE.

An aromatic herb used in cosmetics such as shampoos, rinses and skin fresheners. The white and yellow heads of chamomile flowers are used in cosmetics as coloring agents. (Contains azulene) Used for its skin-soothing quality and to add aroma to cosmetics.

CHOLESTEROL.
An emulsifier and lubricant in various cosmetics. Nontoxic to the skin.

CITRIC ACID.
Used in many cosmetic products as a preservative, and as an emulsifier. Also acts as an astringent and is derived from citrus fruit fermentation.

CLEANSING CREAMS AND LOTIONS.
The purpose of these creams and lotions is to dissolve oil, break up dirt and grime, and allow for easier make-up removal. Three types of cleansing creams with similar ingredients include cold creams, liquefying creams, and washing creams. Cleansing lotions have the same basic properties as the creams, but usually a different mix of ingredients.

COAGULATE.
To clot.

COCOA BUTTER. (Theobroma Oil)
Known to soften and lubricate the skin. A solid fat from the cocoa plant that is used in soaps, creams, lipsticks and other products. May trigger allergic reactions.

COCONUT OIL.
Extracted from coconut kernels, it is used in soaps, shampoos, massage creams and other products for its lathering and cleansing properties. May act as a skin irritant.

COD LIVER OIL.
Used in skin creams and ointments to facilitate healing, this oil is yellowish with a light odor of fish. Contains Vitamins A and D.

COLD CREAM.

A cleansing cream that feels cool when applied to the skin. Usually contains a mixture of mineral oil, beeswax, borax, and water, along with other additives.

COLLAGEN.

A protein substance found in the skin, muscle, bone, and tendon. For cosmetic use, it is often taken from animal tissue and promoted as an anti-wrinkle agent. Topical collagen applied to the skin does no more than other emollients for wrinkle prevention or treatment. Certain emollients without collagen may be even more effective as moisturizers than those containing collagen. Injected directly into the skin collagen is used to minimize certain skin imperfections (e.g. certain fine lines and wrinkles, acne scars, etc.). Collagen fibers are woven together like threads in fabric, providing a network of support to the body and skin.

COMEDO.

A comedo refers to a plug that interferes with the sebaceous gland duct; a clogged pore. A blackhead is an open comedo; a whitehead is closed.

COMEDOGENIC.

A substance having the ability to cause blackheads and whiteheads in those who are susceptible.

CORN MEAL.

Produced from corn cobs and sometimes used as a facial masque base. Also found in some face and bath powders.

CORNSTARCH.

Known for its absorptive and soothing qualities. Found in facial, foot and dusting powders, and bath products. May cause an allergic reaction.

COSMETIC.
A product or substance used to embellish or beautify, to improve appearance.

COSMETICIAN.
An individual trained in the use of cosmetics.

COSMETOLOGIST.
A professional trained in the enhancement of personal beauty.

COTTONSEED OIL.
Extracted from the seeds of the cotton plant, this odorless, light yellow oil is used in creams, soaps, baby creams, nail polish remover and other cosmetic products. May cause allergic reactions.

CRYOTHERAPY.
A form of treatment in which a cold substance is applied directly to the problem area. Examples of cryotherapy include freezing with liquid nitrogen or carbon dioxide.

CUCUMBER EXTRACT.
Used in certain astringents. Feels cool when applied to skin. Some tropical varieties may be irritating to the skin.

CUCUMBER JUICE.
Juice extracted from the cucumber and used as an astringent. Also found in some beauty cream formulas, this nontoxic juice has a pleasant smell and feels cool to the skin.

CURETTAGE.
Removing tissue with a curette.

CURETTE.
An instrument used during the process of curettage —to clean or scrape away tissue.

DEMULCENT.
A soothing substance used to alleviate pain associated with inflamed mucous areas. Ginseng and aloe vera are demulcents.

DEODORANTS.
Retard the growth of microorganisms, to control perspiration odors.

DERMABRASION.
A method of treatment involving a "planer" or abrasive instrument (e.g. brushes, sandpaper, fraises), to sand off layers of skin. Used for removal of acne scars, "farmer-sailor" skin, and for other skin conditions.

DERMIS.
The layer of skin below the epidermis, composed of connective tissue, elastin, collagen, nerves, blood vessels, hair follicles and their sebaceous glands, and sweat glands.

DESICCATE.
To dry out.

DETERGENT.
Cleansing agents produced from chemicals, rather than from fats and oils. Soap is made from natural fats. The toxic strength of a detergent is related to its alkalinity.

DIETHYLENE GLYCOL.
Produced by heating ethylene oxide and glycol. A colorless liquid used as a plasticizer, solvent, and humectant in cosmetic creams. Can be absorbed through the skin.

ELECTRODESICCATION.
Electrosurgical procedure used to destroy and dry out a specified section of tissue.

EMOLLIENTS.
A group of moisturizing agents which include eye creams, hand creams, night creams and other skin creams intended to soften the skin and alleviate the effects of dry, flaky skin. Emollients are known for their ability to coat the skin's outer surface, making it feel and look softer. Dry skin, however, is related to an inadequate supply of water inside the skin. A good emollient may protect the skin against too much loss of moisture.

EMULSIFIERS.
Agents which aid in the production of emulsions. Emulsifiers often found in cosmetic preparations include stearates, sterols, polysorbates, and sulfated alcohols.

EMULSION.
A fluid that is formed from the mixture of two or more nonmixable liquids (e.g. oil and water).

EPHILIS.
Freckle.

ESSENCE.
An extracted substance that retains its basic and most desirable flavor in a concentrated form.

ESSENTIAL OILS.
Known to retain the basic flavor of the plant from which they are extracted. Long used as preservatives, many essential oils are found in fragrances and flavorings; some have antiseptic and germicidal properties as well.

ESTHETICIAN.
A trained professional concerned with various aspects of skin care. May administer facials, act as a make-up artist or provide related skin care services.

ETHANOL. (Ethyl alcohol)
An antibacterial agent found in astringents, nail polish, antiseptics, and other cosmetics.

EUCALYPTUS OIL.
Extracted from leaves of the eucalyptus tree, it is used as a local antiseptic and is found in skin fresheners. May cause allergic reactions.

EYEBROW PENCILS.
Used to fill in thin or narrow brows. Also used as an eye liner. Should not be applied to the eyelids (upper or lower) inside the lashes. Outline carefully below the bottom eyelashes and above the top lashes. Eye irritation can occur if the substance seeps into the eye.

EYE CREAM.
Used to lessen the appearance of wrinkles in this area. Such creams cannot prevent wrinkles but may make them appear less noticeable.

EYELINERS.
Available in pencil, liquid, or pencil-brush form, eyeliners must be applied and removed with care, as they can cause eye irritation.

EYE SHADOW.
The purpose of eye shadow is to provide color to the eyelid and to accentuate and highlight the eyes. All types should be applied and removed with care. May cause eye irritation.

FACE MASQUES.
Refers to any of several types of "masques" applied to the face. The most common types of commercially-marketed masques include clay (usually for oily skin) and gel (usually for dry skin). Various other types of masques may be purchased or home-prepared. Some over-the-counter masques have been known to cause skin irritations and eye problems.

"FARMER - SAILOR" SKIN.
Skin that has been subjected to many years of intense cold, wind, and sun.

FATTY ACIDS.
Mainly used in the manufacturing of soaps and detergents. Important for healthy skin and regular growth. Nontoxic.

FATTY ALCOHOLS.
Alcohols produced from fatty acids and used in creams and lotions. Cetyl and stearyl alcohols help protect skin from moisture evaporation and impart a silky finish to the skin. Lauryl and myristyl alcohols are employed in various creams and detergents. Comedogenicity varies.

FIBROBLAST.
Cells within the dermal layer of skin that produce collagen.

5-FLUOROURACIL.
Applied externally to treat solar keratoses and other indications of sun-damaged skin. Anti-cancer drug.

FORMALDEHYDE.
Found in nail polish and hardeners, soap, and some hair products. It's used in cosmetics as a disinfectant, germicide, defoamer, and preservative. Can be very irritating to the skin. May cause allergic reactions.

FOUNDATION MAKE-UP.
Make-up base used to tone down oily skin and to provide a moisturizing base for dry skin. This product helps conceal blemishes and protects the skin to some degree from outside elements. There are many types of foundation make-up products. Choice of product should depend on skin type and condition.

FREEZING WITH LIQUID NITROGEN. (Cryotherapy)
A dermatological method used mainly to treat keratoses, freckles, and liver spots.

FRAGRANCE.
A pleasant odor or scent.

FULLER'S EARTH.
An absorbent found in facial masques, dusting powder, dry shampoos, soaps, and other products. Also used as a decolorizing agent. Usually nontoxic to the skin.

GINSENG.
Frequently used in oriental medicine. Employed in cosmetics as a demulcent. Obtained from the ginseng plant of the U.S. and Far East.

GLUCOSE GLUTAMATE.
Utilized as a humectant in creams and lotions, it is found in grape and corn sugars, and animal blood.

GLYCERIDES.
A texturizer and emollient in cosmetic creams. Appears to be nontoxic to the skin.

GLYCERIN.
An emollient, humectant, and solvent. Helps maintain moisture in creams. Found in hand creams, lotions, fresheners, cream rouge, and facial masques.

GLYCERYL MONOSTEARATE.
An emulsifier and dispersing agent in cosmetics such as mascara, facial masques, and hand lotions. Nontoxic to the skin.

GLYCERYL STEARATE.
Used primarily as a humectant in cosmetics. Slightly comedogenic.

GRAPE SEED OIL.
Found in many hypoallergenic creams and other cosmetic lubricants.

GUM ARABIC.
Used in cosmetics as an emulsifier, gelling agent, and stabilizer. Found in many facial masques, rouge, powders, and other products. May trigger allergic reactions in susceptible individuals.

GUM KARAYA.
Found in some facial masques, rouge, compact powders, hair sprays, and hand lotions. Known to cause allergic reactions in susceptible individuals, therefore excluded as an ingredient in hypoallergenic products. Its effects on skin are still under study.

GUMS.
Serve as thickening agents in cosmetics. Found in emollient creams, hand creams, rouges, facial powders, bleach creams, etc. Usually nontoxic to the skin, althogh allergic reactions may occur in susceptible individuals.

GUM TRAGACANTH.
An emulsifier in many cosmetics such as mascara, compact powder and rouge, eye make-up, foundation creams, and hand lotions. Known to cause allergic reactions in sensitive skin.

HAND CREAMS AND LOTIONS.
The purpose of these products is to moisturize and soften the skin's surface. Lotions and creams serve as emollients.

HEMATOMA.
A discolored, swollen area caused by blood beneath the skin. Usually a clotted mass of blood.

HEXACHLOROPHENE.
As an antibacterial agent in cosmetics, this substance is found in cold creams, emollients, soaps, facial masques, and skin fresheners. Products containing hexachlorophene have been known to cause various skin reactions.

HONEY
Made by bees from the nectar of flowers, it is used for coloring, flavoring, and as an emollient in cosmetics.

HORMONE CREAMS AND LOTIONS.
Promoted by cosmetic companies as wrinkle prevention formulas, although very limited evidence exists regarding the effectiveness of these products.

HUMECTANT.
A "wetting" agent (e.g. glycerin and sorbitol) used to preserve moisture content in creams and lotions. Found in many facial masques, antiperspirants, hair products, and cosmetic creams.

HYACINTH.
Obtained from the flower and used in various soaps and perfumes, hyacinth juice can act as a skin irritant and may trigger allergic reactions as well.

HYPOALLERGENIC.
This means that the product is less likely to facilitate a reaction in those who may be sensitive to certain allergens used in regular cosmetics. The actual effectiveness of "hypoallergenic" products is still being debated.

ISOPROPYL ALCOHOL.
This substance is used in cosmetics such as hand lotions and hair color products, as an astringent and antibacterial agent

ISOPROPYL MYRISTATE.
Found in foundation make-up, bath products, mascara, and other cosmetics. Comedogenic. Used to facilitate absorption through the skin.

JOJOBA OIL.
A lubricating substance derived from the jojoba bean and found in many cosmetics.

KAOLIN. (China Clay)
Found in some facial masques, emollients, and bath and face powders, to help absorb oil. Usually nontoxic to the skin.

KERATOSES.
Reddish lesions that develop on sun-damaged skin. Usually begin as smooth spots and turn into raised lesions with a rough surface. Occur frequently on areas exposed to sun. Several methods of treatment are available (e.g. cryotherapy, electrodesiccation, etc.).

LACTIC ACID.
Found in some skin fresheners. May irritate the skin if applied in concentrated form.

LANOLIN.
Derived from the oil glands of sheep. An emulsifier and humectant in cosmetics. May be listed under other names such as acetol, waxolan, and lantrol. Known to produce skin flare-ups in susceptible individuals. May act as an allergen. Found in many lipsticks, mascaras, creams and lotions, bath oil, foundation make-up, cold creams, eye creams, and eye shadows.

LANOLIN ALCOHOLS.
Derived from lanolin and used in many creams and lotions. May cause allergic reactions.

LATEX.
Used in facial masques as a coating agent. May trigger skin reactions.

LAURIC ACID.
An ingredient of many vegetable fats, soaps and detergents. Has foaming properties. May be mildly irritating to the skin.

LAURYL ALCOHOL.
Produced from coconut oil. Used in detergents and perfumes. Is foam-producing. A mild irritant.

LAVENDER OIL.
Found in many perfumes, skin fresheners, and powders. May cause allergic reactions.

LECITHIN.
Derived from the Greek word for "egg yolk," it is an emollient and antioxidant in hand creams, lotions, soaps, and hair products. Obtained from eggs and soybeans.

LEMON.
Used in many cosmetics such as astringents, fresheners, skin creams, and cream rinses. May cause allergic reactions.

LENTIGINE.
Dark spots that occur on the skin as a result of prolonged, extensive exposure to sun.

LIMEWATER.
Used as an alkali in facial masques, skin toners, and hair products.

LINOLEIC ACID.
A fatty acid that is used as an emulsifier in cosmetics.

LINSEED OIL.
An oil obtained from flax seed and used in some emollients. Can trigger allergic reactions.

LIP BRUSH/PENCIL.
Used to outline the lips with lipstick.

LIQUEFYING CREAM.
A cleansing agent developed to "liquefy" when applied to the skin.

LIVER SPOT.
Not connected in any way to the liver, these dark spots often occur on the face and back of hands.

MARJORAM OIL.
Found in some perfumes, soaps, and hair products. Can act as a skin irritant and may cause allergic reactions.

MASCARA.
Applied to provide color and thickness to eyelashes. Known to cause eye irritation.

MATTE FINISH MAKE-UP.
Useful in concealing blemishes. A combination of both foundation and powder.

MAYONNAISE.
The salad dressing sometimes used as a conditioner for dry hair and as an ingredient in a facial masque.

MEDICATED MAKE-UP.
Promoted as make-up that conceals blemishes and treats problem skin. May cause allergic reactions.

MELANOCYTE.
This is a cell that creates melanin, the dark pigment found in the skin, retina, and hair. Located in basal layer of epidermis.

MELANOMA.
A tumor of melanocytes which can be benign or malignant. Of the various forms of skin cancer, malignant melanoma is the most dangerous.

MENTHOL.
Used as a mild local anesthetic. Provides cooling sensation to the skin. Derived from peppermint and other mint oils and produced synthetically from thymol. A common ingredient in many cosmetics (e.g. skin fresheners and creams), menthol is nontoxic in low concentrations.

METHYL HEPTINE CARBONATE.
Obtained from castor oil and used in many creams, toilet waters, lipsticks, and other cosmetics. Can cause allergic reactions.

METHYLPARABEN.
Utilized in cosmetics as a preservative and antimicrobial, it is found in many cold creams, eyeliners, and foundation make-up. May cause allergic reactions in those who are sensitive.

METHYL SALICYLATE. (Oil of Wintergreen)
Employed as a disinfectant and local anesthetic in perfumes, mouthwash, and tooth products. Acts as a skin irritant. Also listed under sweet birch or teaberry oil.

MILK.
As a soothing agent, milk is sometimes used in facial masques and as a skin wash. To prevent bacterial development, it should be rinsed thoroughly from the skin.

MINERAL OIL.
Obtained from petroleum and used in cosmetics primarily as a lubricant. Found in various cold creams, cleansing creams, foundation make-up, eye creams, mascara, hand creams, and many other products. Nontoxic, but some products with mineral oil may be comedogenic.

MINK OIL.
As an emollient, it is found in many creams and lotions.

MOISTURIZERS.
These products may contain substances such as mineral oil, lanolin, beeswax, sorbitol, polysorbates, and stearic acid. Helps the skin feel softer and smoother, provides a layer of oil that protects the skin against evaporation of water.

MUDPACKS.
Used by some as a facial treatment. There are no real skin benefits derived from the use of mudpacks.

MUSK.
Derived from the male musk deer and used in perfumes. May cause allergic reactions.

MUSTARD OIL.
Found mainly in soaps, lubricants, and liniments. Strong concentrations may irritate the skin.

MYRISTYL ALCOHOL.
An emollient used in creams and lotions. Gives a smooth texture to cosmetics.

OAT GUM.
Employed in cosmetics as a thickener and stabilizer.

OATMEAL.
Traditionally used in various facial masque preparations. Nontoxic to the skin.

OLEIC ACID.
Derived from animal and vegetable fats and oils. Used in the production of various cosmetics such as soaps, cold creams, and lipsticks. Absorbs into the skin more easily than vegetable oils, and may act as a skin irritant.

OLIVE OIL.
Has skin penetrating properties. Found in emollients, lipsticks, soaps, and massage oils. May act as an allergen.

OXALIC ACID.
Found in freckle and bleaching formulas. A strong skin irritant.

PALM OIL.
Used in making soaps, ointments, liniments, and lubricants. Nontoxic to the skin.

PALMITATE.
Utilized as an oil in cosmetics such as eye creams, cream rouges, bath
and hair products.

PANTHENOL.
Found in creams and hair products. Nontoxic to the skin.

PAPAYA.
Used in organic make-up. Can cause allergic reactions.

PARA-AMINOBENZOIC ACID.
Used in sunburn and sunscreen products. May cause allergic reactions in some people.

PARABEN.
Used as a preservative (Methyl- and propyl-). Also used to destroy
bacteria and fungus. May cause an allergic reaction.

PARAFFIN.
Used in many cosmetics such as cold creams, eye make-up, and
liquefying creams. True paraffin is nontoxic to the skin.

PARSLEY OIL.
Employed as a preservative and flavoring in some cosmetics. May
irritate the skin and cause allergic reactions.

PEANUT OIL.
Used in soaps, hair products, liniments and emollients. Usually
nontoxic to the skin.

PENTASODIUM PENTETATE.
Utilized as an emulsifier, preservative, and dispersing agent in
cleansing creams and lotions. May irritate the skin.

PEPPERMINT OIL.
Used in cosmetics such as eye lotions and toilet waters. Local anti-septic. May be a skin irritant.

PETROLATUM. (Petroleum Jelly, Vasoline)
Yellowish white lubricant found in cold creams, lipsticks, liquefy-ing creams and other cosmetic products. Aids in softening and smoothing the skin, but is more difficult to remove than other emollients. Usually nontoxic, but has been known to cause skin flare-ups in susceptible persons.

pH.
A measure of acidity and alkalinity. A neutral solution such as water has a pH of 7.

PHENOL.
Used in face peels, anesthetics, and disinfectants. Produced from coal tar and can be fatal when absorbed through the skin.

PLACENTA.
Promoted as an additive to remove wrinkles. No evidence is avail-able to support this claim.

POLYGLYCEROL.
Utilized in cosmetic preparations as an emulsifier. Nontoxic to the skin.

POLY-SORBATE (20-85).
Effective as an emulsifier in creams and lotions. Serves as a stabilizer of essential oils. Usually nontoxic.

PORE.
A tiny opening on the skin's surface; leads to a sweat gland.

POTASSIUM CARBONATE.
Found in some shampoos, freckle formulas, and soaps. Is a strong irritant to the skin.

POTASSIUM HYDROXIDE.
May be used as an alkali in some soaps, creams, and rouges. Also used as an emulsifier. May irritate skin.

POTASSIUM STEARATE.
Used in the making of soaps, creams, and lotions. Has defoaming properties. Nontoxic.

POTATO STARCH.
Used as a demulcent in dusting powder and as an emollient in some dry shampoos. Can cause allergic reactions.

POWDER. (Face and Compact)
Purpose of powder is to reduce the appearance of "shiny" skin. Most face and compact powders are harmless to the skin.

PRESERVATIVES.
Used in cosmetic products to prevent chemical change, the development of bacterial formation, and product contamination.

PROGESTERONE.
Corpus luteum hormone produced by the ovaries.

PROPYLENE GLYCOL.
Employed as an emulsifier, wetting agent, and humectant in many cosmetics. Generally nontoxic to the skin.

PROPYLENE GLYCOL LAURATE.
Used as an emulsifier in creams and lotions, and as a stabilizer in essential oils. Can cause allergic reactions in those who are sensitive.

PROPYLENE GLYCOL STEARATE.
Used as a lubricant and emulsifier in creams and lotions. Nontoxic.

PROPYLPARABEN.
A preservative in shampoos, facial masques, foundation creams, and other products.

PROTECTIVE CREAMS.
Creams developed to protect the skin from irritating outside elements.

PYRIDOXINE HCL. (Vitamin B_6)
Soothing and nontoxic when applied to skin.

RESORCINOL.
This substance is used as a preservative, antiseptic, and as a soother for itching skin. Found in some lotions and creams, in acne preparations and other cosmetics. May cause skin irritation in sensitive persons.

RIBOFLAVIN. (Vitamin B_2)
Used in emollients. Nontoxic to skin.

ROSACEA.
A condition of acute redness on the face that usually occurs in the cheek and nose areas. It is often found in combination with telangiectasia and/or acneiform lesions.

ROSE GERANIUM.
Found in some dusting powders and perfume. Can trigger allergic reactions.

ROSEMARY OIL.
Used in perfume, liniments, and hair products. Made from rosemary flowers. Nontoxic to skin.

ROSE OIL.
Employed in toilet waters, perfumes, and ointments. Can cause allergic reactions.

ROSE WATER.
Used to provide a pleasant scent to emollient creams, eye lotions, and other cosmetics. Created through the distillation of fresh flowers.

ROUGE.
Designed to give color to the cheeks. Available in compact, liquid, cream, and dry rouge forms. May irritate the eye area or cause allergic reactions in the hypersensitive.

RUBBING ALCOHOLS.
Utilized in skin fresheners, astringents, and perfumes. May be a skin irritant.

RUBEFACIENTS.
A counterirritant that brings about reddening of the skin.

SAFFLOWER OIL.
May be used in certain lotions and creams as a skin softener. Nontoxic.

SALAD OIL.
Includes the edible vegetable oils. These oils are found in many cosmetic creams, cleansers, lipsticks, and hair products. Nontoxic.

SALICYLIC ACID.
Derived naturally from wintergreen leaves and other plants; made synthetically by combining phenol with carbon dioxide. Found in facial masques, suntan lotions and oils, deodorants, and creams. Acts as a preservative, antimicrobial agent, and skin softener. May cause allergic reactions in susceptible individuals.

SEBACEOUS GLANDS.
Glands that produce sebum.

SESAME OIL.
Found in some emollients, sunscreen products, shampoos, and soaps.

SHARK OIL.
An excellent source of Vitamins A and D, this oil is used in lubricating creams and lotions. Because of its fishy smell, it is usually found in very small quantities in cosmetic preparations.

SILICONES.
Used in hand lotions, protective creams, hair, and nail products, silicones include any number of rubbers, resins, fluid oils and compounds derived from silica. When applied externally there is no known toxicity.

SILK POWDER.
A coloring substance in soaps and facial powders. Can cause allergic reactions.

SKIN FRESHENER.
A toning agent that is often promoted for dry or sensitive skin. Contains less alcohol than astringents. Refreshing and cool when applied to the skin. Skin reactions are rare.

SOAP.
Usually made by mixing caustic alkalies with fatty acids. Sodium salts and fats are commonly used in bar soap; potassium replaces sodium in liquid soaps. Soaps vary in their ingredients, in cleansing strength, and ability to cause irritations. Some soaps can act as irritants and may cause allergic reactions or rashes in those who are sensitive.

SODIUM BORATE.
A preservative and emulsifier in cleansing creams, eye lotions, and hair setting preparations. Tends to dry out the skin and may be an irritant.

SODIUM LAURYL SULFATE.
A wetting agent, emulsifier and detergent in hand lotions, creams, hair products, bubble baths and other cosmetic preparations. Acts as a degreasing agent and may dry or irritate the skin.

SORBITAN STEARATE.
An emulsifying agent in creams and lotions. May also be found in sunscreen preparations, rouge, and antiperspirant deodorants.

SORBITOL.
Primarily used as a humectant in cosmetics. Found in hair sprays, masques, lotions, shampoos, creams, make-up foundation and many more products. Nontoxic when applied to skin.

SOY GLYCERIDE.
An emollient found in soaps, shampoos and bath products.

SPERMACETI. (Cetyl Palmitate)
A waxy substance derived from the sperm whale that is found in many creams and ointments. It is an emollient in cleansing creams and it is also found in cold creams and shampoos (to enhance their gloss and thicken the products). Usually nontoxic, but occasionally causes irritation.

STABILIZER.
In cosmetics, an ingredient added to a product to provide body and maintain texture.

STEARIC ACID.
Widely used in cosmetic preparations such as creams, soaps, deodorants, ointments, and foundation make-up. A pearlish white fatty acid that may act as an allergen in sensitive individuals.

STEARYL ALCOHOL.
An ingredient in creams, ointments, and some hair products. Adds texture; has antifoaming properties. (May be produced from sperm whale oil.) Generally nontoxic.

STEROL.
Includes various solid alcohols from plants and animals. Acts as a lubricant in creams and lotions, hair products, and hand care formulas. Nontoxic.

SUBCUTANEOUS.
Directly beneath the skin.

SUNFLOWER SEED OIL.
A soft yellow oil containing high concentrations of Vitamin E. Used as a lubricant in soaps.

SURFACTANT.
A substance that eases contact between the skin and cosmetic preparations. Includes wetting agents, emulsifiers, and dispersing agents.

SWEET ALMOND OIL.
Common ingredient in perfumes, emollients, and fine soaps. Nontoxic to skin.

TELANGIECTASIA.
Small dilated blood vessels that form a network of reddish-purple lines on the skin. Sometimes called "spiders" because of the appearance of the condition.

TEXTURIZER.
A substance that upgrades the texture of cosmetics. Helps to smooth out a formula or provide a desired level of thickness.

TITANIUM DIOXIDE.
Utilized in creams, powders, eye make-up, and other cosmetics to protect against solar rays and external irritations.

TOCOPHEROLS. (Vitamin E)
Used as an antioxidant in cosmetics. When applied topically, Vitamin E may act as an allergen or cause skin rashes.

TOILET SOAP.
Consists primarily of pure soap manufactured from high quality substances.

TRANSLUCENT POWDER.
Similar in composition to other face powders, except that translucent powder contains higher levels of titanium dioxide. More opaque than other such powders.

TRICHLOROACETIC ACID.
Used topically as part of the acid face peel procedure. May cause allergic reactions.

TRICHLOROETHANE.
A solvent with anesthetic and degreasing properties. Can penetrate the skin and cause eye and skin irritations.

TRICLOCARBAN. (TCC)
Used in soaps, cleansing agents, and medicated cosmetics as an antiseptic and to destroy bacteria. Nontoxic.

TRIDECYL ALCOHOL.
An emulsifying chemical in lipsticks, creams, and lotions. Nontoxic.

TRIETHANOLAMINE STEARATE.
A moisture-absorbing agent and oil emulsifier, used in making creams, fragrances, masacara, and liquid make-ups. Can cause skin irritation.

TRIOLEIN. (Glyceryl Trioleate)
Olein. Found in various fats and oils and used to make cosmetic creams and oils. Nontoxic.

TURTLE OIL.
May be used in emollients and nail products. Promoted as an extra special ingredient, but there is no scientific evidence to suggest that it is any better than other oils.

UREA.
Used in various moisturizers as a humectant. Secreted through sweat glands. Also produced synthetically.

VEGETABLE GUMS.
Serve to thicken and cream cosmetic products. May cause allergic reactions in those who are sensitive.

VEGETABLE OILS.
Widely used in cleansing and moisturizing creams, powders, lipsticks, and other cosmetics. Also found in "hypoallergenic" formulas. Derived from sesame, peanut, olive, corn, and other plants. Nontoxic.

VITAMIN A.
Utilized in creams and oils. A substance that can be absorbed through the skin.

VITAMIN E.
See "tocopherols".

WITCH HAZEL EXTRACT.
A local anesthetic, astringent, and skin freshener. It is 70-80% alcohol.

XERODERMA.
Refers to dry skin.

ZINC OXIDE.

A white, powdery mineral used in powders, foundation creams, face packs, rouge, white eye shadow, bleach/freckle creams and other products. It is also used in ointments to sooth burns and other skin irritations, as an antiseptic and protective agent in various skin diseases.

ZINC SULFATE.

The result of zinc and sulfuric acid combined. A crystalline salt found in skin tonics, astringents, and other cosmetics. May irritae the skin.

ZYDERM COLLAGEN IMPLANT.

A form of collagen produced from calf hide, injected into skin to minimize the appearance of skin imperfections such as acne scars, post-surgical and traumatic scars, fine creases around the eyes and lip area, some frown and smile lines.

Index